PSORIASIS - TYPES, CAUSES AND MEDICATION

Edited by **Hermenio Lima**

Psoriasis - Types, Causes and Medication
http://dx.doi.org/10.5772/56549
Edited by Hermenio Lima

Contributors

Sibel Dogan, Nilgün Atakan, Hermenio C Lima, Robyn S. Fallen, Anupam Mitra, Laura Morrissey, Sebastiano Bucolo, Valerio Torre, Giuseppe Romano, Filippo Farri, Maura Filidoro, Claudio Caldarelli, Carmelo Quattrocchi, Hani A. Al-Shobaili, Muhammad Ghaus Qureshi, Farideh Zafari Zangeneh, Fatemeh Shooshtary, Delia Colombo

Published by InTech

Janeza Trdine 9, 51000 Rijeka, Croatia

Publishing Process Manager Ana Pantar
Technical Editor InTech DTP team
Cover InTech Design team

Additional hard copies can be obtained from orders@intechopen.com

Psoriasis - Types, Causes and Medication, Edited by Hermenio Lima
p. cm.
ISBN 978-953-51-1065-1

For EU product safety concerns:
IN TECH d.o.o., Prolaz Marije Krucifikse Kozulić 3, 51000 Rijeka, Croatia,
info@intechopen.com or visit our website at intechopen.com.

Meet the editor

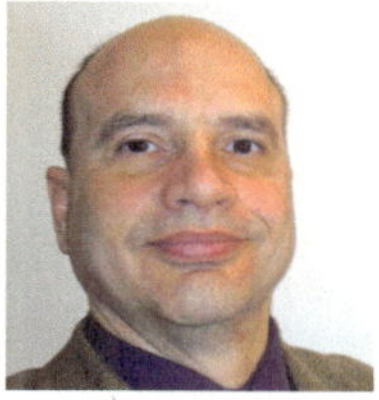

Dr. Hermenio C. Lima is a Clinical Immunologist and Dermatologist. He finished Medical School at the Federal University of Ceará (Brazil) in 1989. He received a PhD (Doctor of Science – DSc) in Tropical Public Health with major in Immunology at Harvard School of Public Health (USA) in 1990. Currently, he is Associate Clinical Professor at Division of Dermatology, Department of Medicine, Michael G. DeGroote School of Medicine at McMaster University (Canada). He received a Teaching Award as voted by the Michael G. DeGroote School of Medicine Class of 2012. Dr. Lima published 61 articles in peer-reviewed specialized journals, and has 677 citations in Google Scholar. His h-index is 14 (2013).

Contents

Preface

By virtue of the dynamic nature of the scientific process, the description of the type, pathogenesis and treatment of a disease is always a work in progress. Each day new research shapes and refines our understanding of disease processes; an attempt to describe the current scientific understanding provides merely a snapshot of a body of knowledge that is constantly changing. However, characterizing a disease using homeostatic and physiological terms allows the creation of a framework to convey the most up-to-date theories while maintaining the potential for their evolution.

The complex nature of any disease can similarly be unveiled through understanding the historical context of our current understanding, examining prevailing hypotheses and extrapolating horizons for new research. To develop a framework for understanding of psoriasis and its evolution, the first perception to be changed is the prevalent teleological view of pathogenesis. The general notion that psoriasis is one disease with one mechanism must be changed. This model full of logic and consequences does not apply in many other areas of medical and non-medical science. However, the belief that certain phenomena are best explained in terms of purpose rather than cause infest the medical scientific field. As such, it is necessary to move to a new approach to describing the relationship among immune system, other systems and environment.

For better development of this book about psoriasis, the main objective was to provide insights on the types, causes, and treatments of this prevalent humans disease. Any successful program of knowledge transference has to discuss the pivotal role of some of these aspects of immunopathophysiology, how our understanding of its mechanism evolved, and how to block or revert the effect of a specific immunological disequilibrium. Through this, the aim is to explain some facts of modern science that might be useful for clinicians to understand the basis of psoriasis. Moreover, an important goal is to dispel some misinformation that might have a negative impact on the use of new immunomodulators and medications available. Treatment basis and therapeutic response experience strongly supports the use of immunomodulators as important modalities in the treatment of many diseases in all fields of medicine. Studies with these therapeutic agents, which act in different steps of the inflammatory cascade, have also shown significant efficacy in psoriasis.

This approach might substantially improve the transference of disease knowledge for physicians and is intended to improve the quality of medical services that endorses training of excellence and assesses the qualifications of physicians, most of whom will be naïve to clinical dermatological practices.

Enjoy the book.

Hermenio Lima, MD PhD
McMaster University, Canada

Section 1

Types of Psoriasis

Chapter 1

Psoriasis — Types, Causes and Medication

F.Z. Zangeneh and F.S. Shooshtary

Additional information is available at the end of the chapter

http://dx.doi.org/10.5772/54728

1. Introduction

Although the skin disease psoriasis was first recognized as a distinct disease as early as 1808 [1], its pathogenic mechanisms have eluded investigators for decades, its definition by Ferdinand von Hebra as a distinct entity dates back only to the year 1841 and estimates of its prevalence around 2-3% of the general population, and is characterized by an exaggerated proliferation of keratinocytes secondary to an activated immune system. The incidence is highest at the age of 20–39 years in males and 40–59 years in females, with an equal male-to-female ratio [2]. Psoriasis clinically manifests as raised, well defined erythematous plaques with irregular borders and silvery scales, affecting the upper and lower extremities equally, but with a predilection for the elbows, knees, scalp, and trunk. Psoriasis vulgaris or plaque psoriasis accounts for almost 90% of the dermatological presentation of the disease, but several other forms, including guttate, inverse, erythrodermal, pustular, and palmoplantar psoriasis may occur, as well as nail involvement. Psoriasis may have significant systemic involvement, which is underscored by the coexistence of various clinical disorders, including eye, cardio-vascular, and intestinal problems, metabolic syndrome, and joint inflammation. It has a very high negative impact on quality of life, requires long-term treatment which usually has a high social and economic impact and is also associated with a decreased life span [3] [4].

2. Psoriasis types

Psoriasis classification

No one classification of psoriasis satisfies all the mentioned requirements. Usually, criteria are intermingled (Table 1), and subclasses are nonexclusive. Similar problems exist with the clinical classification of psoriatic arthropathy [5].

Morphologic aspects of elementary lesions	Pustular, non-pustular but also plaque, nummular, guttate, gyrate, rupioid, elephantine, ostraceous, etc.
Degree of inflammation	Mainly inflammatory vs mainly hyperkeratotic
Pattern distribution	Extensory, inverse, seborrhoeic, widespread
Extent	One site (scalp, nail, etc.), many sites, generalized
Time of first onset	Early vs late onset
Velocity of propagation	Stable, unstable, eruptive

Table 1. Features which have been considered in different classifications of psoriasis [6]

Classification criteria based on purported etiology rank higher in formalization compared with purely morphological ones.

2.1. Classifying psoriasis: The spectrum of clinical varieties

Psoriasis, a papulosquamous skin disease, has several different types, including: **psoriasis vulgaris** (common type), **guttate psoriasis** (small, drop like spots), **inverse psoriasis** (in the folds like of the underarms, navel, and buttocks), and **pustular psoriasis** (pus-filled, yellowish, small blisters). When the palms and the soles are involved, this is known as **palmoplantar psoriasis**.

2.2. Psoriasis vulgaris (chronic stationary psoriasis, plaque-like psoriasis)

The commonest type of psoriasis, accounting for 90% of all cases, is psoriasis vulgaris, in which papulosquamous plaques are well-delineated from surrounding normal skin. The plaques are red or salmon pink in color, covered by white or silvery scales and may be thick, thin, large or small (Figure 1). They are most active at the edge: rapidly progressing lesions may be annular, with normal skin in the centre. Plaques are usually distributed symmetrically, and occur most commonly on the extensor aspects of elbows and knees; scalp (where they rarely encroach beyond the hairline), lumbosacral region, and umbilicus. Active inflammatory psoriasis is characterized by the Koebner phenomenon, in which new lesions develop at sites of trauma or pressure [7].

2.2.1. Classification of psoriasis vulgaris according to phenotype: plaque-type psoriasis

There is also variation of features of psoriasis dependent on anatomical sites. Until the reasons for this variation are fully understood, they are proposed to be recorded as a phenotypic entity, although subsequently they may be shown to be part of a common pathogenetic mechanism. A further distinction arises according to the age of onset of plaque psoriasis [8]. Henseler and Christophers are credited with identifying two ages of onset: type I occurring at or before the age of 40 years—this accounts for approximately 75% of patients; and typeII presenting after the age of 40 years, with a distinct peak at 55–60 years [9].

http://dx.doi.org/10.5772/54728

2.2.2. *Plaque-type psoriasis: Chronic plaque psoriasis*

As a consequence, chronic plaque psoriasis is the form of the disease entered into clinical trials and the object of the majority of investigations of genetics and pathogenesis of psoriasis. It is characterized by red, scaly, discoid lesions varying in size from 0.5 cm in diameter to large confluent areas on the trunk and limbs (Figure 1). There is a sharp line of demarcation between a plaque and clinically normal, uninvolved skin. Longitudinal studies of individual plaques have demonstrated that plaques are dynamic [10] with an active and expanding edge, sometimes to the extent that the advancing edge may become annular (Figure. 2) leaving clinically normal skin in the centre of the original plaque. The variety of plaque is characterized by well-demarcated plaques with a loosely adherent silvery-white scale, which preferentially affect the elbows, knees, lumbosacral area, intergluteal cleft, and scalp. Occasionally, pustular lesions may appear in the plaque (so-called psoriasis with pustules). Chronic plaque psoriasis is the most common variety of psoriasis representing about 70% to 80% of psoriatic patients [11].

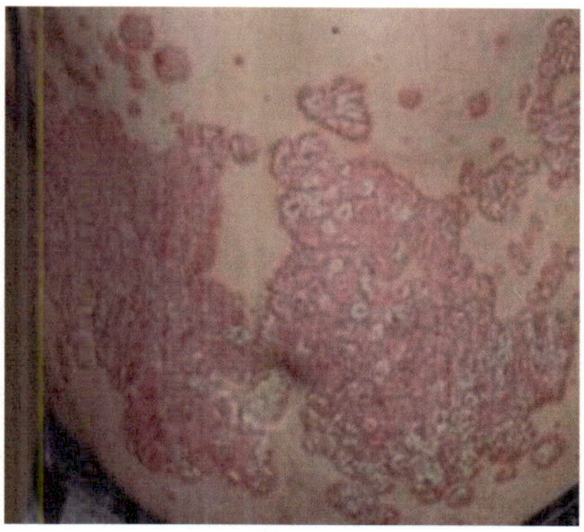

Figure 1. Typical plaque of Psoriasis Vulgaris.

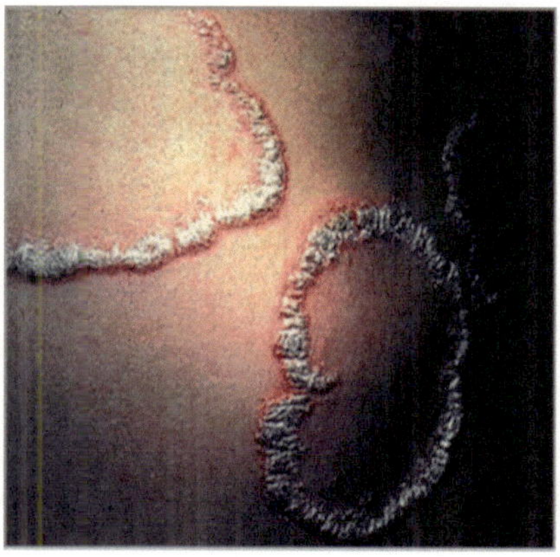

Figure 2. Annular psoriasis showing clearance in centre of plaque.

Under the heading of plaque psoriasis, it is proposed to include, as subdivisions, a new, more logical nomenclature of phenotypes associated with specific anatomical sites, distribution, size and thickness of plaques [8].

2.2.3. *Site-specific variants of Psoriasis Vulgaris (PV)*

Site-specific variants of psoriasis vulgaris exist. Flexural (inverse) psoriasis in intertriginous sites is shiny, red, and typically devoid of scales (figure 3); sebopsoriasis, which can be confused with seborrhoeic dermatitis, has greasy scales and occurs in eyebrows, nasolabial folds, and postauricular and presternal sites. Psoriasis vulgaris will probably prove to be several closely related but phenotypically and genotypically distinct conditions [8].

Flexural/intertriginous: Inverse psoriasis (Flexural Psoriasis or Psoriasis of the Skin Folds) is usually located in the skin folds: i.e. armpits, under the breasts, skin folds around the groin and between the buttocks. It is particularly subject to irritation from rubbing and sweating because of its location in skin folds and tender areas (Figure 3). Plaques are thin, have minimal scale and a shiny (nonscaly) surface commonly accompanied by secondary fissuring and/or maceration. The major clinical manifestation of inverse psoriasis is sharply demarcated erythematous plaques, with varying degrees of infiltration, which often tend to itch and burn [12]. The most common lesions are found in inguinal, submammary, interglutaeal, umbilicus and genital folds, whereas the popliteus and axillae are rarely involved. The humidity and heat typical of these sites, together with the combination of local traumatic factors often associated with infections caused by dermatophytes and Candida albicans, together contribute to the development of psoriasis in accordance with the Koebner phenomenon. The Koebner phenomenon is an indicator of disease activity, may have a prognostic value, and is associated with early onset of psoriasis [13]. The Koebner phenomenon was first described by Heinrich Koebner (1838–1904) and refers to the fact that in people with certain skin diseases, especially psoriasis, trauma is followed by new lesions in the traumatized but otherwise normal skin, and these new lesions are clinically and histopathologically identical to those in the diseased skin [14].

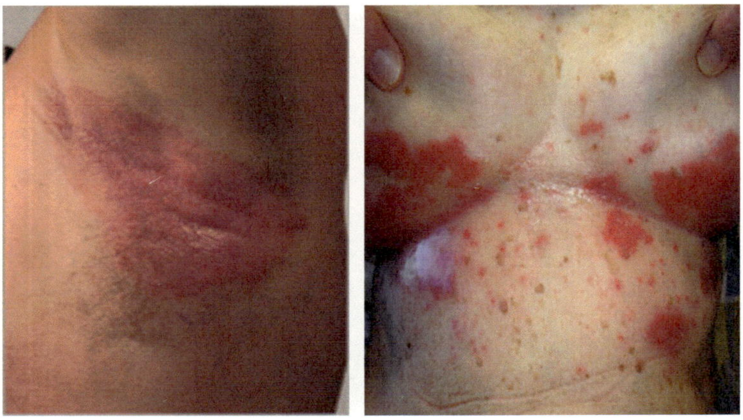

Figure 3. Flexural psoriasis, notes the relative lack of scale.

http://dx.doi.org/10.5772/54728

Seborrhoeic: Seborrhoeic psoriasis ('sebopsoriasis'), so called because of its similarity in morphology and anatomical distribution to seborrhoeic dermatitis, may occur either in isolation or associated with plaque psoriasis elsewhere. Sites of involvement are the nasolabial folds (Figure 4), medial cheeks, nose, ears, eyebrows, hair line, scalp, presternal and interscapular regions. Characteristically the lesions are thin, red and well-demarcated (somewhat like intertriginous psoriasis) with variable degrees of scaling.

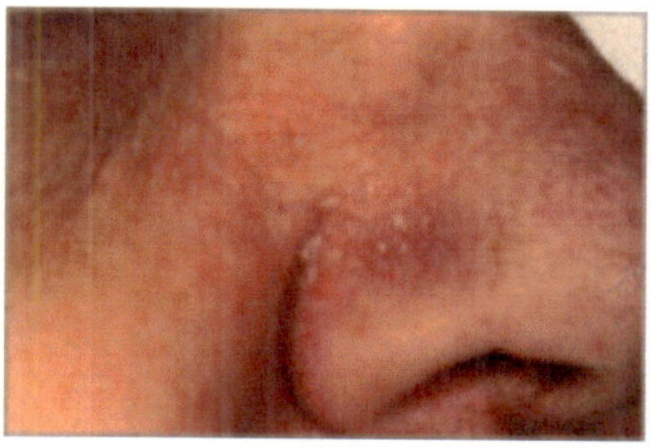

Figure 4. Seborrhoeic psoriasis, nasolabial, 'greasy' appearance and finely scaled.

Scalp: The scalp is frequently the site of initial presentation and is the commonest anatomical site to be involved by psoriasis. Morphologies range from discrete plaques to total scalp involvement with either thick plaques or scaly nonthickened areas almost identical to seborrhoeic dermatitis. Sites of predilection include the immediate postauricular area and occiput. An important and fascinating observation is that the scalp lesions rarely extend > 2 cm beyond the hairline. Compared with psoriasis elsewhere, scalp involvement is frequently asymmetrical (Figure 5).

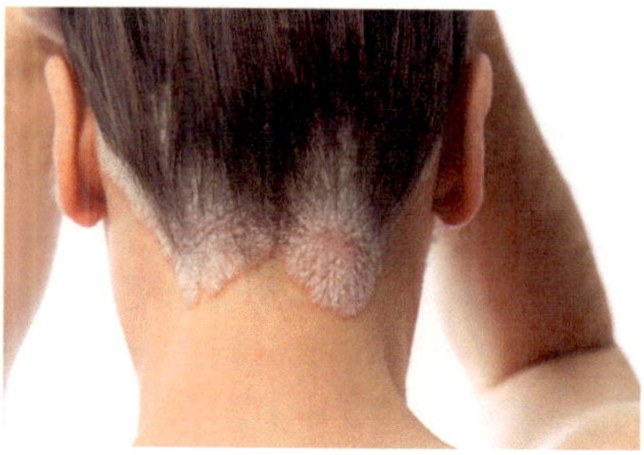

Figure 5. Psoriasis of the scalp.

Palms/soles (nonpustular): Palmoplantar pustulosis, consisting of yellow-brown, sterile pustules on palms and soles, is still described in textbooks of dermatology as a subtype of psoriasis. About 25% of people with palmoplantar pustulosis also have chronic plaque psoriasis. The disease has different demographics to psoriasis vulgaris in that patients are predominantly women (9:1 female: male ratio) and either current or previous smokers (95%) and onset occurs in the 4th or 5th decades of life (Figure 6) [15].

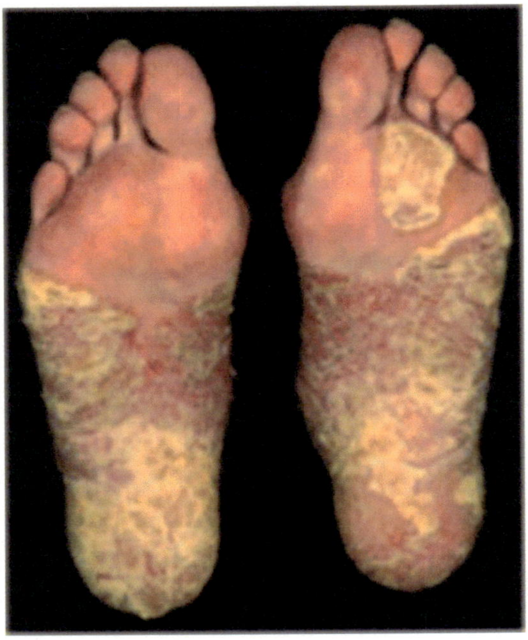

Figure 6. Plantar involvement by plaque psoriasis.

2.3. Guttate psoriasis

Psoriasis affects approximately 2% of the world population, and of these cases, 2% manifest as guttate psoriasis [16]. Guttate means "drop" in Latin; aka Teardrop Psoriasis, Raindrop Psoriasis or Psoriasis Exanthematic) is the second most common type of psoriasis. Guttate psoriasis (GP), an important clinical variant, most frequently occurs in adolescents and young adults. It is characterized by the sudden onset of widely dispersed small red scaly plaques mainly over the trunk and proximal limbs. The symptoms of GP are numerous small, red, drop-like spots which cover a large portion of the skin. Spots have an abundant scaling. Lesions are usually located on the trunk, arms, legs and scalp. GP can clear up without treatment or disappear and resurface in the form of plaque psoriasis. GP is especially common in children or young adults with a family history of psoriasis and follows streptococcal infection and/or acute stressful life events [17]. Guttate flares in patients with established psoriasis vulgaris (PV) are also frequently observed. These observations, taken together with investigative studies, indicate an important pathogenetic link between GP and PV [15]. GP is often associated with a preceding streptococcal throat infection or a rise in anti-streptococcal serum titer [16] [18]. Bacterial streptococcal infections (strep throat, chronic tonsillitis) or a viral respiratory infection usually precede and trigger the first signs of Guttate Psoriasis in persons predisposed to psoriasis. Herein, Dr. Loh in 2012 reports a case that suggests such an association. This 15-year-old girl presented with a case of acute guttate psoriasis shortly after the onset of mono-nucleosis. The structural characteristics of her eruption and her skin biopsy findings are consistent with guttate psoriasis (Figure 7).

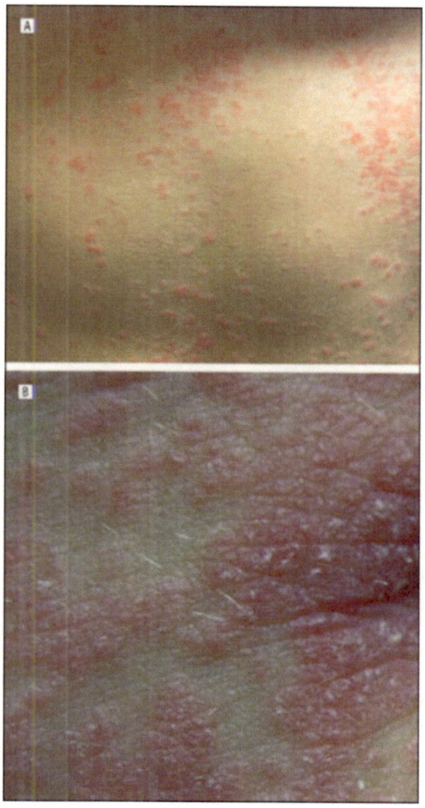

Figure 7. Clinical photographs of the abdomen w th guttate psoriasiform papules and plaques. A,Unmagnified image. B, Image at higher unspecified magnification [19].

2.4. Pustular psoriasis: In a population survey of psoriasis, pustular lesions were reported at any time during the course of psoriasis by about 20% of patients [11]

Generalized pustular psoriasis: Patients with generalized pustular psoriasis (GPP) may have preexisting plaque psoriasis or develop it after pustular episodes. Acute episodes may be triggered in patients with plaque psoriasis by irritating topical therapy or abrupt corticosteroid withdrawal [20]. At the onset of an attack of acute GPP (von Zumbusch type) the skin becomes very red and tender. There may be fever and systemic symptoms such as anorexia and nausea. Within hours, myriads of pinhead-sized pustules appear, studding the erythematous background (Figure 8). Pustules may become confluent, producing lakes of pus. Subsequently, the pustules dry out, and the skin peels off, leaving a glazed, smooth erythematous surface on which new crops of pustules may appear [21]. GPP should be distinguished from acute generalized exanthematic pustulosis, a self-limiting febrile drug reaction usually resolving in 2 weeks after withdrawal of the suspected agent, characterized by pinpoint nonfollicular pustules on erythematous patches mainly involving folds. Single necrotic cells in the epidermis, eosinophils, and vasculitic changes in the dermis are peculiar pathologic features [22] [23].

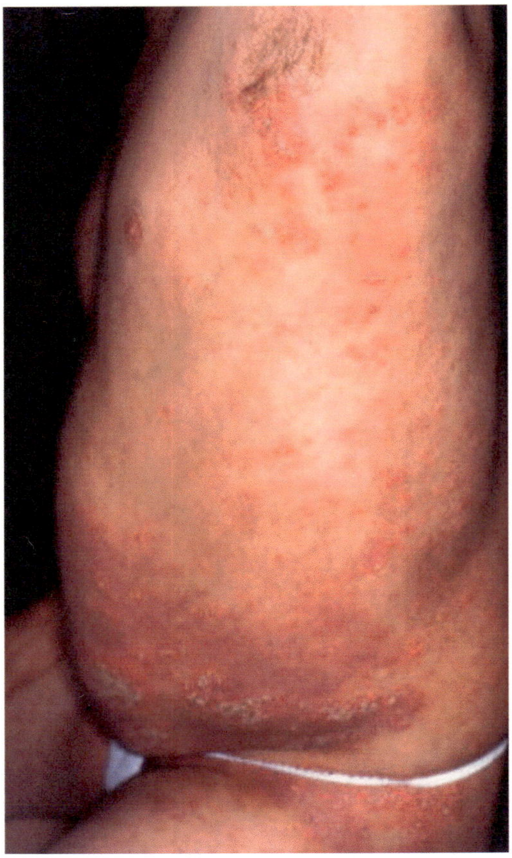

Figure 8. Early phase of generalized pustular psoriasis with edematous plaques and pustules.

Localized pustular psoriasis: Besides so-called psoriasis with pustules (sometimes referred to by the misleading term "localized form of generalized pustular psoriasis"), 2 main clinical varieties are reported as localized pustular psoriasis: acrodermatitis continua of Hallopeau and palmoplantar pustulosis.

Acrodermatitis continua, also known as dermatitis repens, is a rare, chronic, pustular eruption of the fingers and toes (Figure 9). Often, it begins after a localized trauma starting at the tip of a single digit [24].

Palmoplantar pustulosis: is characterized by hyperkeratosis and clusters of pustules over the ventral aspects of hands and/or feet (Figure 10). Classification of palmoplantar pustulosis within the spectrum of psoriasis is controversial. The disease predominates in women (more than 70% of patients are women) and is much more strongly associated with smoking than plaque psoriasis [25]. Palomar-plantar pustulosis (PPP) generally appears between the ages of 20 and 60. PPP causes large pustules to form at the base of the thumb or on the sides of the heel. In time, the pustules turn brown and peel. The disease usually becomes much less active for a while after peeling.

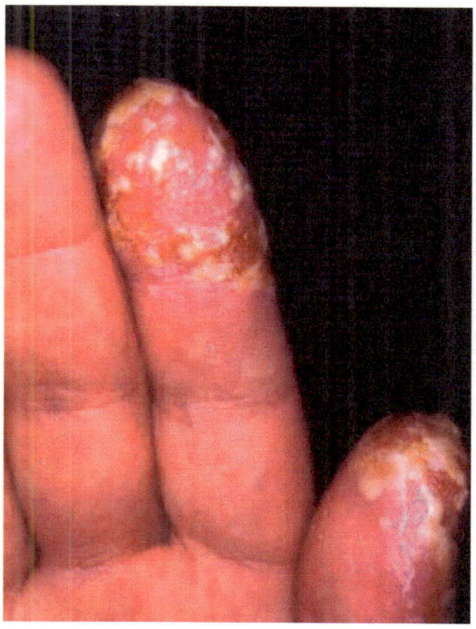

Figure 9. Acrodermatitis continua showing crops of pustular lesions at the tips of the fingers.

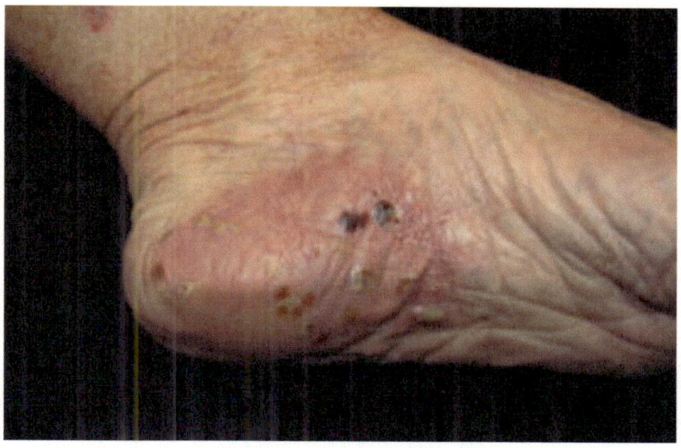

Figure 10. Palmoplantar pustulosis.

2.5. Erythrodermic psoriasis

As already mentioned, plaque psoriasis is a rather stable disorder. The transition to a more extensive involvement, due to frequently unidentifiable triggering factors, is frequently marked by the onset of an inflammatory phase with predominant erythema and limited scaling associated with itching and rapidly progressing lesions. This unstable psoriasis may sometimes evolve to whole-body involvement. The erythrodermic phase is dominated by generalized erythema, loss of peculiar clinical features of psoriasis, and skin failure, that is, inability to maintain homeostatic functions [26]. Erythrodermic psoriasis characterized by severe scaling, itching, and pain that affects most of the body, erythrodermic psoriasis disrupts the body's chemical balance and can cause severe illness (Figure11). This particularly inflammatory form of psoriasis can be the first sign of the disease, but often develops in patients with a history of plaque psoriasis.

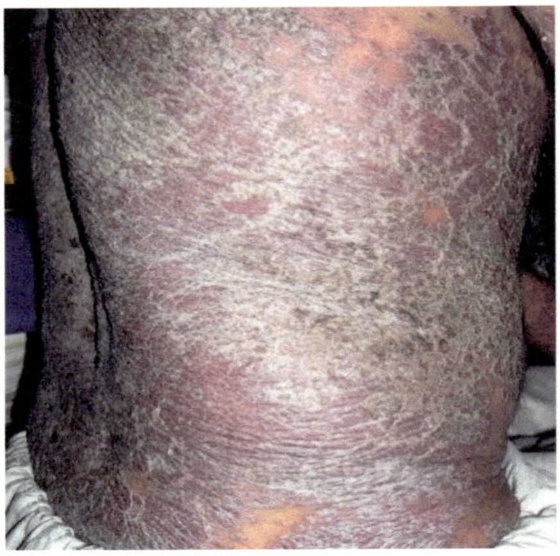

Figure 11. Erythrodermic psoriasis.

2.6. Nail psoriasis

Approximately 50% of all patients with psoriasis develop characteristic nail changes as a clinical correlate of psoriatic inflammation of the nail matrix and/or nail bed. The most frequent signs of nail psoriasis are pitting and distal onycholysis [27]. Clinical manifestations range from pitting, yellowish discoloration, and paronychia, to subungual hyperkeratosis, onycholysis, and severe onychodystrophy (Figure 12) [28].

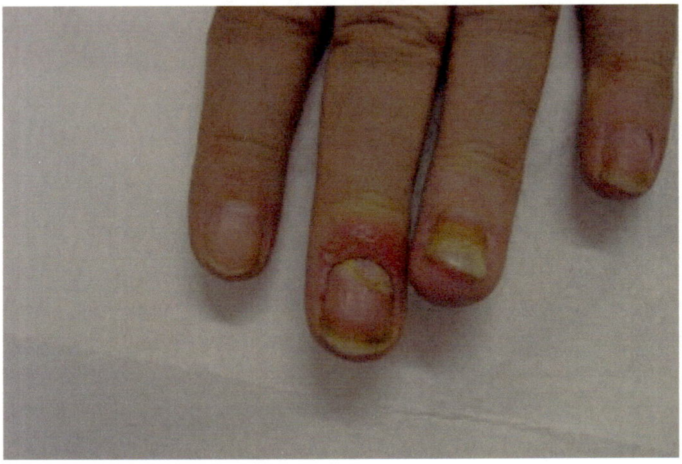

Figure 12. Yellowish discoloration of fingernails.

http://dx.doi.org/10.5772/54728

2.7. Psoriatic arthritis

Psoriatic arthritis (PsA) is a chronic inflammatory joint disease occurring in 6–39 % of patients with psoriasis with a prevalence of PsA in the general population of about 0.1–0.25 % [29] [30]. Based on the several common clinical and radiological features, PsA is considered as a member of the family of spondyloarthritides [31]. This type of arthritis can be slow to develop and mild or it can develop rapidly. PsA can be a severe form of arthritis with prognosis similar to that of rheumatoid arthritis (RA) [32]. Psoriatic arthritis (PsA) is characterized by focal bone erosions mediated by osteoclasts at the bone–pannus junction. Importantly, 80% of patients with psoriatic arthritis have nail psoriasis (Figure13) [33]. Recognition of bone as an active organ that interacts with its environment is a relatively new development. In the pathogenesis of bone destruction associated with rheumatoid arthritis, the synovium is a site of active interplay between immune and bone cells. The interaction between T cells and osteoclasts is a critical issue in the field of osteoimmunology [34]. Further differentiate mechanisms of bone resorption and repair in PsA and RA and likely will uncover additional therapeutic targets [35].

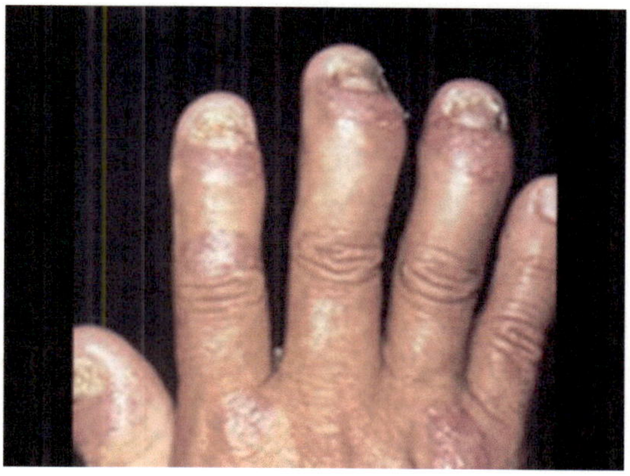

Figure 13. Psoriatic arthritis hand changes over time.

3. Pesoriasis causes

Psoriasis – Pathogenesis

Today, psoriasis is recognized as the most prevalent autoimmune disease caused by inappropriate activation of the cellular immune system. There are two main hypotheses about the process that occurs in the development of Psoriasis. The first considers psoriasis as primarily a disorder of excessive growth and reproduction of skin cells. The problem is simply seen as a fault of the epidermis and its keratinocytes and is characterized by hyperproliferation with incomplete differentiation of epidermal keratinocytes and decreased keratinocyte apoptosis. The second hypothesis sees the disease as being an immune-mediated disorder (immunosuppressant medications can clear psoriasis plaques) in which the excessive reproduction of skin cells is secondary to factors produced by the immune system. T cells become active, migrate to the dermis and trigger the release of cytokines which cause inflammation and the rapid production of skin cells. It is not known what initiates the activation of the T cells. That work initially pointed towards a major role of T lymphocytes as inducers of the disease phenotype and the pathogenic contribution of this cell type has now been tested through clinical studies of more than a dozen immune modifying biological agents in patients with psoriasis. The inflammatory cytokines such as tumor necrosis factor (TNF) are likely to play major pathogenic roles in this disease and that other types of inflammatory leucocytes may also serve key pathogenic functions. Here we will review some recent works on psoriasis that advances our overall understanding of disease pathophysiology regarding neuroendocrine immunology. The concept of Psoriasis & Supersystems considers site of recognition, skin barrier in the sympathetic nervous (beta2 adenoceptors) and immune systems.

Psoriasis & supersystems

The brain and the immune system, or the "supersystems", a term recently coined by Tada (1997), are the two major adaptive systems of the body [36]. Although the immune system has been often regarded as autonomous, the last two to three decades provided strong evidence that the central nervous system (CNS) receives messages from the immune system and vice versa messages from the brain modulate immune functions. Thus, the brain and the immune system are involved in functionally relevant cross-talk, whose main function is to maintain homeostasis [37]. In psoriasis it seems that the most important components of these supersystems are ß2 adenoceptors and tumor necrosis factor alpha (TNFα). Recent studies show that the ß2-adrenergic receptor is specifically associated with the homeostasis of skin barrier. Ca has critical role in this function. Increasing evidences indicate that TNF may have immunosuppressive effects, since long-term exposure to TNF can directly prevent the activation of T cells. ß2-adrenergic receptor interacts with TNFα which is evaluated in below, respectively.

3.1. Skin's barrier function

3.1.1. Homeostasis of skin barrier: Self-referential system

The skin barrier homeostatic function is a self-referential system because it is always monitoring its original function, i.e., water impermeability. This function is regulated by the peripheral function [38]. Epidermal homeostasis is understood as the maintenance of epidermal tissue structure and function by a fine tuned regulatory mechanism balancing proliferation and cell loss by desquamation and apoptosis [39]. Stem cells of the basal layer or stratum basal in the epidermis have a crucial role in maintaining tissue homeostasis by providing new cells to replace those that are constantly lost during tissue turnover or following injury [40]. cAMP and calcium influence the formation and maintenance of barrier function [41].

3.1.2. Skin: An indispensable and protective barrier

The first protective barrier is provided by the skin, our largest organ. It serves as the interface between the organism and the outside world and it serves many functions, such as the retention of body fluids, maintenance of body temperature, and protection against UV-light, chemical influxes, wounds, and the invasion of micro-organisms. The protective barrier function is performed by the keratinocytes of the epidermis, which are continuously produced by proliferating stem cells of the basal layer or stratum basal and differentiate during a 14 day journey towards the surface [42].

3.1.3. Skin: Epidermal barrier capacity (lipid/protein polymer structure)

Stratum corneum (SC) & Ceramides (family of lipid molecules)

Epidermal barrier capacity is controlled by lipids that fill the extracellular space of the skin's surface layer-the stratum corneum. Lipid synthesis for skin barrier function takes place within the keratinocytes in all nucleated epidermal layers. Lipids are stored within the epidermal lamellar bodies (secretory organells) or keratinosomes, which are ultrastructurally visible at the level of the upper spinous layer and in the granular layer. In the outermost granular layer, the contents of lamellar bodies are secreted into the intercellular domains of the stratum granulosom–stratum corneum interface. Lamellar bodies mainly contain phospholipids, glucosylceramides and cholesterol as well as hydrolytic enzymes, which convert phospholipids, glucosylceramides and sphingomyelinase to free fatty acids and ceramides. Then, lamellar bodies cause in the formation of an impermeable, lipid-containing membrane that serves as a water barrier and is required for correct skin barrier function. The Stratum Corneom (SC) contains three types of lipids -- ceramides, cholesterol and free fatty acids. These lipids have different chemical compositions and different functions throughout the body. There are nine different types of ceramides in the Stratum Corneom, conveniently named ceramide 1 through ceramide 9, and they account for 40-50% of the lipids in this outermost layer. A ceramide is composed of sphingosine and a fatty acid. Ceramides are found in high concentrations within the cell membrane of cells. They are one of the component lipids that make up sphingomyelin, one of the major lipids in the lipid bilayer. Ceramide can actually act as a signaling molecule. The most well-known functions of ceramides as cellular signals include regulating the differentiation, proliferation, programmed cell death (PCD), and apoptosis (Type I PCD) of cells [43].The proliferation rate of keratinocytes to corneocytes is matched by the shedding of old corneocytes at the SC [44] and skin tissue maintains a steady number of SC layers regardless of age [45].

Desquamation, the process of cell shedding from the surface of the stratum corneum, balances proliferating keratinocytes that form in the stratum basale. These cells migrate through the epidermis towards the surface in a journey that takes approximately fourteen days. During cornification, the process whereby living keratinocytes are transformed into non-living corneocytes, the cell membrane is replaced by a layer of ceramides which become covalently linked to an envelope of structural proteins (the cornified envelope). This complex surrounds cells in the stratum corneum and contributes to the skin's barrier function [41]. SC serves as the principal barrier against the percutaneous penetration of chemicals and microbes and is capable of withstanding mechanical forces [46].

Stratum corneum (SC) & Proteases (kallikrein family of serine proteases)

Interestingly, two major proteases of stratum corneum SCCE/KLK7/hK7 and SCTE/KLK5/hK5 together can destroy three major components of the corneodesmosomes: DSC1, DSG1 and CDSN [47]. These enzymes belong to kallikrein family of serine proteases. Their expression starts in suprabasal keratinocytes where their inactive precursors undergo a processing by an unidentified trypsin-like protease [48]. In stratum corneum, these enzymes appear in the intercellular spaces suggesting their involvement in the desquamation [49]. Recent discoveries have highlighted the importance of various proteases, protease-inhibitors, and protease targets as key players in epidermal barrier function [50]. It has become clear in recent years that serine proteases have an important role in epidermal homeostasis, and the signaling cascades are gradually being identified [41].

3.1.4. Skin: Epidermal proteases

The specific differentiation program in stratified skin requires a specialized proteolytic system to detach the corneocytes from each other without causing a barrier defect. A number of different proteases have been reported to be involved in the desquamation process and to contribute to the barrier function of the skin. Based on their proteolytic domain, proteases are classified into serine, threonine, cysteine, aspertate, metallo, and glutamate proteases. Especially serine proteases (SPs) seem to be involved in epidermal permeability barrier homeostasis as it was reported that SP activity was increased after acute barrier disruption and that blockade by topical SP inhibitors accelerated barrier recovery after acute abrogation [51].

3.1.5. Skin: Adherent junction proteins (Epidermal junction)

The Epidermal junction (EJ) plays a crucial role in the formation and maintenance of epithelial and endothelial barriers. The EJ is a complex basement membrane synthesised by basal keratinocytes and dermal fibroblasts. It plays a fundamental role as a mechanical support for the adhesion of the epidermis to the dermis and regulates the exchanges of metabolic products between these two compartments; besides, it serves as a support for keratinocytes migration during wound healing, and is traversed by various cell types (LC, lymphocytes...) during immunologic and inflammatory processes [52]. Basal keratinocytes are connected to adjacent cells by several types of intercellular junctions (including gap and adherens junctions), the most characteristic of which are the desmosomes. Formation of adherens junctions and desmosomes requires extracellular calcium [53].

Summary 1: Psoriasis & skin's barrier function

Although the Psoriasis is a multifactorial disease, the studies show that disruption the homeostasis in skin's barrier is the main factor. Several factors interfere of hemostatic establishment in skin. 1) Heterogeneous Structure (lipid/protein) of this barrier that is the main cause of hemostasis. This two compartment structures is renewed continuously and when the barrier function is damaged, it is repaired immediately. 2) Several proteases important for desquamation (skin shedding). 3) The Epidermal junction (EJ) plays a crucial role in the formation and maintenance of epithelial and endothelial barriers. Formation of adherens junctions and desmosomes requires extracellular calcium. Raising the calcium concentration in the cell culture medium from 0.05 to 1.2mM [53] stimulates keratinocytes to form strong cell-cell adhesions in vitro. 4) In epidermal keratinocytes, both extracellular and intracellular Ca++ is reported to be important to cell differentiation and proliferation.

3.2. Skin's sympathetic fibers: Neuroendocrin regulation

The skin is a complex organ containing afferent and efferent neural networks, glands, blood vessels, smooth muscle elements, connective tissues and immune cells, many of which are modulated by catecholamines and glucocorticoid hormones. Glucocorticoids and catecholamines reach skin tissues as circulating hormones and catecholamines are released in skin by projections of the sympathetic nervous system. The sympathetic division of the autonomic nervous system within the skin is supplied by postganglionic fibers of the paravertebral chain ganglia. Catecholamines also are produced locally by keratinocytes [54] [55].

3.2.1. Skin's Beta2 adrenergic receptors (β-ARs)

Beta2 adrenergic receptors were identified in keratinocytes more than 30 years ago, but their function in the epidermis continues to be elucidated [56]. The β-adrenergic (β-ARs) agonists are capable of modulating the two distinct components of keratinocyte directional migration via divergent signaling pathways: 1) migration rate via a cAMP-independent, mitogen-activated-protein-kinase-dependent pathway [57] and 2) galvanotaxis by a cAMP-dependent one. Previous data have shown that both endogenous and exogenous catecholamines act to attenuate the permeability response to various inflammatory mediators via β1- [58] and β2-adrenoceptors [59] [60] [61] [62]. Additionally, because β-adrenergic agonists and antagonists modulate both keratinocyte migration and galvanotaxis, they could be valuable tools for controlling reepithelialization and restoration of barrier function, an essential component of the wound healing process.

3.2.2. β-ARs signaling cascade

In skin, it has been proposed that epinephrine activates keratinocyte beta2AR to modulate calcium influx and begin the differentiation cascade crucial to the native architecture of the epidermis [54]. The beta2AR desensitizes upon repeated activation through several mechanisms, including downregulation of the number of beta2AR receptors [63] [64]. Indeed, beta2AR expression is more highly expressed at the basal layers of the epidermis and decreases in expression toward the stratum corneum [54], suggesting that epinephrine may be activating the receptor to increase intracellular calcium levels and induce differentiation.

3.2.3. β2 adrenergic receptor (β-ARs): Phosphodiesterase

The cyclic nucleotide phosphodiesterases comprise a group of enzymes that degrade the phosphodiester bond in the second messenger molecules cAMP and cGMP. They regulate the localization, duration, and amplitude of cyclic nucleotide signaling within subcellular domains. The PDE superfamily of enzymes is classified into 11 families, namely PDE1-PDE11, in mammals. PDEs have different substrate specificities. Some are cAMP-selective hydrolases (PDE4, 7 and 8); others are cGMP-selective (PDE5, 6, and 9). A phosphodiesterase type 4 inhibitor, commonly referred to as a PDE4 inhibitor, is a drug used to block the degradative action of phosphodiesterase 4 (PDE4) on cyclic adenosine monophosphate (cAMP). It is a member of the larger family of PDE inhibitors. The PDE4 family of enzymes is the most prevalent PDE in immune cells. They are predominantly responsible for hydrolyzing cAMP within both immune cells and cells in the central nervous system [65]. Since the late 1980s, PDE4 inhibitors have been under investigation as anti-inflammatory therapies against asthma and chronic obstructive pulmonary disease. Due to the broad anti-inflammatory activity of PDE4 inhibitors, their possible use in the treatment of atopic dermatitis and psoriasis was examined.

3.2.4. β2 adrenergic receptor (β-ARs): cAMP & Calcium

In psoriasis, keratinocytes within the psoriatic lesions demonstrate a low cAMP response to ß2-AR activation [66]. These findings point to a role for the cutaneous ß2-AR network in maintaining epidermal function and integrity. Moreover, it has also been shown that ß2-AR density in the human epidermis depends on the calcium concentration [67] [54], where undifferentiated keratinocytes express approximately 7500 AR per cell and differentiated keratinocytes express only 2500 receptors underlining an important function for the 2-AR in the differentiation process in human skin [68]. Stimulation of the beta2-AR leads to a transient increase in the keratinocyte intracellular calcium concentration [69] [70] and this likely occurs through several signaling cascades. The mean increase in intracellular calcium of psoriatic keratinocytes was significantly reduced compared with control keratinocytes when intracellular calcium stores were mobilized from endoplasmic reticulum with thapsigargin (an inhibitor of the endoplasmic reticulum Ca2+ ATPase was used to empty the Ca2+ stores from endoplasmic reticulum) [71].

Summary 2: Psoriasis & β2 adrenergic receptor (β-ARs)

It has already been established that the skin is an important peripheral neuro-endocrine-immune organ that is tightly networked to central regulatory systems. These capabilities contribute to the maintenance of peripheral homeostasis. Skin cells and skin as an organ coordinate and/or regulate not only peripheral but also global homeostasis. Activation of the sympathetic system is the most common studied in literature, but other possibilities have to be considered, like impairment of epidermal barrier function, which is already described. ß2-AR density in the human epidermis depends on the calcium concentration and calcium plays an important part in the regulation of proliferation and differentiation of keratinocytes.

3.3. Skin's immunity function: Keratinocytes as immune sentinels

Keratinocytes can sense pathogens and mediate immune responses to discriminate between harmless commensal organisms and harmful pathogens. Keratinocytes are continuously in contact with external stimuli and have the capacity to produce several soluble mediators. Pathogen-associated molecular patterns (PAMPs) are recognized, among others, by Toll-like receptors (TLRs). Epidermal keratinocytes express several TLRs, located either on the cell surface (TLR1, TLR2, TLR4, TLR5 and TLR6) or in endosomes (TLR3 and TLR9) [72]. Keratinocytes are also an important source of chemokines and express chemokine receptors, and therefore can modulate an immune response by attracting different cell types into the skin.

3.3.1. Keratinocytes as a secretory organ of cytokines

Keratinocytes produce a wide array of cytokines, including tumor necrosis factor and interleukin 1α (IL-1α), IL-1β, and IL-6. Disruption of the permeability barrier increases the expression of these cytokines [73] [74]. Studies in mice deficient in these cytokines or their receptors have shown delays in permeability barrier recovery after acute disruption, suggesting that the increased cytokine production facilitates barrier repair [75] [76]. Cytokines are well known to stimulate lipid synthesis and metabolism, and one could anticipate that an increase in epidermal lipids induced by cytokines could facilitate lamellar body formation and permeability barrier recovery [75] [77] [78].

3.3.2. Sympathetic regulation of innate immunity

Activation of the sympathetic nervous system (noradrenergic nerves and adrenal medulla) exerts a potent anti-inflammatory action upon the innate immune system. Adaptive immune cells are known to express primarily the β2AR, while innate immune cells appear to express the β2AR, a1AR, and a2AR. In the case of adaptive immune responses, however, signals from the brain are transmitted back to the periphery, primarily via activation of the HPA and the SNS [79]. The magnitude of an adaptive immune response appears to be regulated by the release of norepinephrine within the direct vicinity of activated CD4+ T cells and B cells located within lymphoid tissue. The released norepinephrine stimulates the β2AR expressed on the immune cells to regulate the level of gene activity. The immune cell self-regulated immune response develops and progresses normally with the participation of norepinephrine to regulate the level of the response in an attempt to maintain immune homeostasis [80]. The importance of sympathetic nervous system has been studied in skin disorders. In vitiligo, there is a dysregulation of catecholamine biosynthesis with increased plasma and epidermal noradrenaline levels associated with high numbers of β2-ARs in differentiating keratinocytes and with a defective calcium uptake in both keratinocytes and melanocytes. In atopic eczema, a point mutation in the β-AR gene could alter the structure and function of the receptor, thereby leading to a low density of receptors on both keratinocytes and peripheral blood lymphocytes [81]. In psoriasis, β-ARs are downregulated, because the increased circulating levels of catecholamines have been observed in psoriatic patients [82] [83] [84] and a 10-fold increase in the expression of the Phenylethanolamine N-methyltransferase (PNMT), the epinephrine sythetic enzyme is also found in basal keratinocytes in involved psoriatic epidermis [85]. It is tempting to propose that long-term exposure to increased levels of catecholamines, in the circulation or locally derived by the keratinocytes themselves, in combination with increased desensitization of beta 2AR in individuals, may predispose to psoriasis. Cathecolamines regulate the immune system at regional, local and systemic levels via adrenergic receptors expressed on immune cells [86] and interestingly, β-AR blockers may cause this inflammatory autoimmune skin disease [87] [88].

3.3.3. Psoriasis & immune system

Psoriasis is a chronic inflammatory, immune-mediated skin disease, which affects 2%-3% of the population worldwide [89]. Psoriasis was until recently regarded as a T-cell-driven disease with presumed (auto) immune mechanisms as its primary cause [90] [91].

3.3.4. Psoriasis & the innate immune system

The innate immune system provides the first line of defense against infection by detecting the presence of invading pathogens in a non-specific manner. Cells of the innate immune system include macrophages, dendritic cell (DC), monocytes, neutrophils, mast cells, natural killer (NK), NKT cells and $\gamma\delta$ T cells. Innate immune cells recruit additional leukocytes to the site of inflammation by releasing cytokines and chemokines. Many innate immune cells can also directly kill invading pathogens. In addition, the innate immune system plays a crucial role in the initiation and direction of the adaptive immune response. Mechanisms regulating barrier integrity and innate immune responses in the epidermis are important for the maintenance of skin immune homeostasis and the pathogenesis of inflammatory skin diseases [92].

3.3.5. Is psoriasis a result of the bidirectional communication between the nervous and immune systems?

The existence of an association between the brain and immunity has been documented. Data show that the nervous and immune systems communicate with one another to maintain immune homeostasis. Activated immune cells secrete cytokines that influence central nervous system activity, which in turn, activates output through the peripheral nervous system to regulate the level of immune cell activity and the subsequent magnitude of an immune response. One key mechanism responsible for such coordination involves the autonomic nervous system (norepinephrine), which serves as the messenger from the mind to the body for all organ systems, including the immune system [93]. The antigen-activated immune system regulates CNS activity through the release of cytokines that bind to receptors located peripherally on the vagus nerve or sympathetic nerve terminals or centrally within the CNS or at the blood-brain barrier. Subsequently, the CNS communicates back to the immune system by activating the SNS or the HPA to release the neurotransmitter norepinephrine or a corticosteroid hormone, respectively. Lymphocytes express receptors that bind norepinephrine and corticosteroids, providing a mechanism for these ligands to activate intracellular signaling pathways, which regulate the level of immune cell activity. A bidirectional communication between the nervous and immune systems is to maintain homeostasis, whether this requires an increase or decrease in immune cell activity. Also, skin-brain axis fMRI studies on patients with psoriasis have revealed that the processing of facial expressions of disgust is significantly impaired in subjects with psoriasis as compared with normal controls in that blood flow in the anterior insular cortex is reduced. This appears to be a coping mechanism [94].

Summary 3: Psoriasis & neural immunoregulation

The brain and the immune system are the two major adaptive systems of the body. During an immune response the brain and the immune system "talk to each other" and this process is essential for maintaining homeostasis. Two major pathway systems are involved in this cross-talk: the hypothalamic-pituitary-adrenal (HPA) axis and the sympathetic nervous system (SNS). This overview focuses on the role of SNS in neuroimmune interactions, an area that has received much less attention than the role of HPA axis. Evidence accumulated over the last 20 years suggests that norepinephrine (NE) fulfills the criteria for neurotransmitter/neuromodulator in lymphoid organs. The immune cell self-regulated immune response develops and progresses normally with the participation of norepinephrine to regulate the level of the response in an attempt to maintain immune homeostasis. Cathecolamines regulate the immune system at regional, local and systemic levels via adrenergic receptors expressed on immune cells.

3.4. Psoriasis comorbidities: Overactivity of sympathetic nervous system

The more common comorbidities include psoriatic arthritis and anxiety/depression disorder [95] [96]. More recently, psoriasis has also been reported to be associated with metabolic disorders including obesity, dyslipidaemia and diabetes [97] [98]. Moreover, an increased mortality from cardiovascular disease in patients with severe psoriasis has been documented, and psoriasis may confer an independent risk of myocardial infarction especially in young patients [99].

3.4.1. Psoriasis & metabolic syndrome

Recent studies of epinephrine stimulation at the β2 adrenergic receptor reveal important potential long-term beneficial effects in the metabolic syndrome [100]. The association between psoriasis and metabolic disorders such as obesity, dyslipidemia, and type 2 diabetes has shown that severe psoriasis might be associated with increased mortality rate due to cardiovascular disorders [97] [98] [101].

3.4.2. Psoriasis & cardiovascular disease

The study by Gelfand et al. in 2006 indicated that patients with psoriasis are more likely than the general population to have diabetes, high cholesterol, and other "traditional" risk factors for heart disease [99] [102]. Recent studies suggest that psoriasis, particularly if severe, may be an independent risk factor for atherosclerosis, myocardial infarction (MI), and stroke. Mehta et al. in 2010 conducted a cohort study using the General Practice Research Database to determine if severe psoriasis patients have an increased risk of cardiovascular (CV) mortality [103].

3.4.3. Shared risk factors

The existence of shared risk factors between psoriasis and both CV and metabolic conditions has been shown in several epidemiological studies which demonstrate that the same comorbidities are present in psoriasis patients, regardless of age or ethnicity [104] [105].

Summary 4: Conclusive remarks

This review shows that the overactivity of sympathetic nervous system occurs in Psoriasis disease. Abnormalities of β-ARs in their expression, signaling pathway, or in the generation of endogenous catecholamine agonists by keratinocytes have been implicated in the pathogenesis of cutaneous diseases such as atopic dermatitis, vitiligo and psoriasis. These studies suggest that mainly the localization of Beta2-adrenergic receptors in the epidermis and play an important part in the calcium dynamics and barrier homeostasis of epidermal keratinocytes [106].The decrease expression of beta2 adrenergic receptor mRNA in involved psoriatic epidermis shown by RT-PCR [107]. Together, these findings suggest that the downregulation of the number of beta adrenergic receptors, rather than an inherent defect in the receptor itself, is the mechanism that is responsible for the reduced beta-adrenergic responsiveness seen in psoriatic epidermis. This decreased response to endogenous agonists then results in a decrease in intracellular cAMP and thus an increase in keratinocyte proliferation. This downregulation can be about overactivity of sympathetic nervous system. Polimorphism studie show that inactivity of Beta2 adrenoceptor is the main cause in this disorder. Beta2 antagonists wreck this condition and reduction of cAMP could cause disruption in skin barrier hemostasis. Freund et al. in 2012 have used boron-based molecules to create novel, competitive, reversible inhibitors of phosphodiesterase 4 (PDE4). The co-crystal structure reveals a binding configuration which is unique compared to classical catechol PDE4 inhibitors, with boron binding to the activated water in the bimetal center. These phenoxybenzoxaboroles can be optimized to generate submicromolar potency enzyme inhibitors, which inhibit TNF-α, IL-2, IFN-γ, IL-5 and IL-10 activities in vitro and show safety and efficacy for topical treatment of human psoriasis [108]. However, it may be that currently utilized therapies also work by modifying this signaling pathway. For example, vitamin D, currently used as a topical treatment of psoriasis, has been shown to increase the generation of cAMP in response to betaAR agonists [109] Glucocorticoids, the mainstay of topical therapy for psoriasis, increase both the expression of beta2AR in keratinocytes, and the generation of cAMP in response to agonists [110]. UVB irradiation, another mainstay in the treatment of psoriasis, has been shown to increase beta2AR-mediated cAMP accumulation [111].

4. Psoriasis — Medication

Psoriasis is skin disease with unknown etiology. There is no cure for psoriasis, but there are many treatments that can decrease the symptoms and appearance of the disease.

Treatment options

In general, there are three treatment options for patients with psoriasis: Phototherapy, topical and systemic. A combination of therapies is often recommended. Combining various topical, systemic and light treatments often allows lower doses of each and can result in increased effectiveness.

4.1. Topical treatment: Topical drugs

First line management of adult mild-to-moderate adult plaque psoriasis is with topical treatment, including vitamin D analogues and topical corticosteroids. Topical therapies are indicated for patients whose affected area is < 10% of the body surface area (BSA). Topical vitamin D analogues (VD) and topical steroids (TS) are both widely used topical treatments for psoriasis. Calcipotriol is a vitamin D analogue that regulates epidermal cell proliferation and differentiation, as well as production and release of pro-inflammatory cytokines. TS present a wide range of biological effects such as inhibition of the recruitment and migration of inflammatory cells, modulation of cytokine synthesis, chemokines release and regulation of DNA synthesis [112].Topical corticosteroids are available in different potencies and formulations but despite more than 40 years of experience, their use remains mostly based on individual experience. Published guidelines often specify the place of topical steroids within psoriasis treatment strategies [113] [114] [115] but not the efficacy and practical modalities of use. It should be noted that the majority of adverse events seen with topical therapies are cutaneous rather than systemic in nature and that the risk–benefit ratio for these patients is better with topical therapies than with biological [116].

4.2. Light therapy (phototherapy)

Solar ultraviolet (UV) radiation has been used since ancient times to treat various diseases. This has a scientific background in the fact that a large number of molecules (chromophores) in different layers of the skin interact with and absorb UV. These interactions may have both positive and negative biological implications. Most of the positive effects of solar radiation are mediated via ultraviolet-B (UVB) induced production of vitamin D in skin [117]. In our day's phototherapy is a valuable option in the treatment of many psoriatic and nonpsoriatic conditions, including atopic dermatitis, sclerosing skin conditions such as morphea, scleroderma, vitiligo, and mycosis fungoides [118]. UVB radiation reaches the epidermis and the upper dermis where it is absorbed by DNA, trans-urocanic acid (trans-UCA), and cell membranes [119]. Absorption of UVB by nucleotides leads to the formation of DNA photoproducts, primarily pyrimidine dimers. UVB exposure reduces the rate of DNA synthesis. In addition, UVB radiation causes photoisomerization of trans-UCA to cis-UCA which has immunosuppressive effects. Furthermore, UV radiation can affect extranuclear molecular targets (cell surface receptors, kinases, phosphatases, and transcription factors) located in the cytoplasm and in the cell membanes [119]. Keratinocytes, circulating and cutaneous T lymphocytes, monocytes, Langerhans cell, mast cells and fibroblasts are all targeted by narrowband UVB [119]. Narrowband UVB induces also local and systemic immunosuppressive effects which may particularly contribute to the beneficial effects of this light source. UVA radiation penetrates more deeply into the skin than UVB, and reaches not only epidermis, but also dermis with blood vessels affecting dermal dendritic cells, dermal fibroblasts, endothelial cells, mast cells, and granulocytes [120]. UVA radiation is absorbed by pyridine nucleotides (NAD and NADP), riboflavins, porphyrins, pteridines, cobalamins and bilirubin [120] Porphyrins and riboflavins are photosensitizers. UVA effects are dominated by indirect DNA damage caused by reactive oxygen species such as singlet oxygen. The ability of UVA radiation to cause skin erythema is approximately 103 to 104 times lower than that of UVB. As UVA-1 is even less erythematogenic than broadband UVA much higher doses of UVA-1 can be tolerated by the patients. UVA-1 phototherapy works mainly through induction of apoptosis of skin infiltrating T cells, T-cell depletion and induction of collagenase-1 expression in human dermal fibroblast [121] [122].

Sunlight: Already several thousands of years ago sunlight (heliotherapy) was used to treat a variety of skin conditions in Egypt, Greece and Rome [123]. Ultraviolet (UV) light is a wavelength of light in a range too short for the human eye to see.

UVB phototherapy: Controlled doses of UVB light from an artificial light source may improve mild to moderate psoriasis symptoms. UVB phototherapy, also called broadband UVB, can be used to treat single patches, widespread psoriasis and psoriasis that resist topical treatments.

Narrowband UVB therapy: A newer type of psoriasis treatment, narrowband UVB therapy may be more effective than broadband UVB treatment. It's usually administered two or three times a week until the skin improves, then maintenance may require only weekly sessions.

Goeckerman therapy: The combination of UVB treatment and coal tar treatment is known as Goeckerman treatment. The two therapies together are more effective than either alone because coal tar makes skin more receptive to UVB light.

Photochemotherapy: Photochemotherapy involves taking a light-sensitizing medication (psoralen) before exposure to UVA light. UVA light penetrates deeper into the skin than does UVB light and psoralen makes the skin more responsive to UVA exposure.

Excimer laser: This form of light therapy, used for mild to moderate psoriasis, treats only the involved skin. A controlled beam of UVB light of a specific wavelength is directed to the psoriasis plaques to control scaling and inflammation. Healthy skin surrounding the patches isn't harmed.

Pulsed dye laser: Similar to the excimer laser, the pulsed dye laser uses a different form of light to destroy the tiny blood vessels that contribute to psoriasis plaques.

Systemic treatment: Oral or injected medications

Patients with moderate to severe disease generally require systemic agents (e.g. cyclosporin, methotrexate, oral retinoids, fumaric acid esters) to control their disease adequately. The severity of psoriasis traditionally has been evaluated by objective measurement of the extent of the body surface affected and consideration of the subtype of psoriasis, degree of disability, and feasibility of topical therapy [124].

Retinoids: Several systemic retinoids (derivatives of vitamin A) have been developed for the treatment of psoriasis. Systemic retinoids are known to have immunosuppressive and anti-inflammatory activity and to modulate epidermal proliferation and differentiation [125]. As mentioned previously, clinical data suggest that combination retinoid–PUVA therapy may be more effective than either treatment alone, and may minimize the toxicities associated with each modality through dose-sparing or independent chemopreventive effects [126] [127].

Methotrexate (MTX): It was introduced as a therapy for psoriasis in 1958 (Edmomudson et al., 1958). Taken orally, methotrexate helps psoriasis by decreasing the production of skin cells and suppressing inflammation. It may also slow the progression of psoriatic arthritis in some people. Methotrexate is generally well tolerated in low doses. Hepatic fibrosis typically occurs after total cumulative MTX doses of at least1.5 g. [128]. The risk of hepatotoxicity may decrease if MTX is given in short courses and rapidly discontinued after clinical improvement [129].

Cyclosporine: It was first used (inadvertently) for the treatment of psoriasis in 1979 [130]. Cyclosporine suppresses the immune system and is similar to methotrexate in effectiveness. Major toxicities associated with cyclosporin therapy include nephrotoxicity, hypertension and immunosuppression

Fumaric acid esters (FAE): Oral FAE therapy for psoriasis was first reported in 1959. Dimethylfumarate, and its metabolite monomethylfumarate, appear to be the principal active components of Fumaderm®. Treatment with dimethylfumarate and/or monomethylfumarate produces a beneficial shift towards Th2-like cytokine secretion associated with a reduction in peripheral lymphocytes (primarily T cells) [131] and inhibits the proliferation of epidermal keratinocytes in patients with psoriasis. Haematological changes, notably leucopenia, lymphopenia and eosinophilia, are frequently observed during FAE therapy [132].

Tumour necrosis factor alpha (TNFα) inhibitors: It is known that TNF alpha is elevated in both the skin and synovium of psoriatic patients and the effectiveness of its blockade by these two agents in psoriasis and Psoriatic arthritis (PsA) confirms its role in their pathogenesis. TNFi (infliximab, etanercept and adalimumab) revolutionised the treatment of autoimmune diseases such as rheumatoid arthritis (RA), ankylosing spondylitis (AS), Crohn's disease (CD) and plaque psoriasis. Anti-TNF alpha therapy has proved to have disease-reducing activity in PsA and psoriasis and appears to be well tolerated [133]. The widespread use of TNFalpha antagonists in recent years has led to the recognition of paradoxical adverse effects, defined as the onset or exacerbation of disorders that are usually improved by TNFalpha antagonists [134]. During these treatments, cutaneous adverse effects may occur like eczema, lupus, alopecia areata or psoriasis, which represents a paradoxical adverse effect.Then, therapy with TNF α inhibitors can be associated with paradoxical reactions. They are considered a class effect of these drugs, and their incidence ranges from 1 to 5%, with paradoxical psoriasis (psoriasis vulgaris, palmoplantar pustulosis, scalp psoriasis and their combinations) being most frequently reported [135].

Phosphodiestrase inhibitors: Phosphodiesterases play a pivotal role in degrading cyclic nucleotides (cGMP, cAMP), key second messengers in all cells. Particularly cAMP plays an important regulatory role in virtually all the cell types involved in the pathophysiology of allergic and inflammatory diseases including asthma and chronic obstructive pulmonary disease, but also skin diseases including atopic dermatitis and psoriasis. Of the cAMP-degrading PDEs, PDE4 is the one that has been studied most extensively in recent years. PDE4 is abundant, and is the major cAMP-degrading isoenzyme in almost all inflammatory and immune cells. In spite of varied structurallasses, highly selective PDE4 inhibitors have the same quality in suppressing several pro-inflammatory mechanisms likecytokine generation and secretion, superoxide generation, degranulation, IgE production, proliferation, histamine generation and chemotaxis [136] [137]. The PDE4 family comprises four genetically distinct subtypes (PDE4 A-D). These subtypes differ with respect to their regulatory behaviour and tissue expression patterns. The search for selective inhibitors of PDE4 as novel anti-inflammatory drugs has continued for more than 30 years and almost two decades have passed since targeting PDE4 became a focus in the development of novel therapeutics for pulmonary inflammatory diseases. The development of PDE4 inhibitors with PDE4B selectivity has been considered a promising approach because much evidence demonstrates that ablation or inhibition of PDE4B produces a broad spectrum of anti-inflammatory effects while minimizing unwanted side effects [138] [139]. Nazarian et al.'s studies in 2009 showed that AN-2728 (PDE4) is well tolerated and demonstrates significant effects on markers of efficacy, with results that were comparable to positive controls. AN-2728 appears to have good therapeutic potential, although further and larger trials are required to assess the long-term safety and characterize the broad utility of this drug [140]. Nevertheless, the impact of PDE4B-selective inhibitors on inflammatory diseases awaits further clinical trials. Several PDE4B and PDE4D selective inhibitors have been designed and synthesized, and their effects on inflammation are under investigation. Although several compounds have demonstrated therapeutic effects in diseases such as asthma, COPD, atopic dermatitis and psoriasis, none have reached the market. A persistent challenge in the development of PDE4 inhibitors has been drug-induced gastrointestinal adverse effects, such as nausea. Despite the challenges and complications that have been encountered during the development of PDE4 inhibitors, these drugs may provide a genuinely novel class of anti-inflammatory agents, and there are several compounds in development that could fulfill that promise [141]. McCann et al., in 2012 showed oral Apremilast targets PDE4 inhibitor, modulates a wide array of inflammatory mediators involved in psoriasis and psoriatic arthritis, including decreases in the expression of inducible nitric oxide synthase, TNF-α, and interleukin (IL)-23 and increases IL-10. In phase II studies of subjects with psoriasis and psoriatic arthritis, apremilast reversed features of the inflammatory pathophysiology in skin and joints and significantly reduces clinical symptoms. The use of an oral targeted PDE4 inhibitor for chronic inflammatory diseases, like psoriasis and psoriatic arthritis, represents a novel treatment approach that does not target any single mediator, but rather focuses on restoring a balance of pro-inflammatory and anti-inflammatory signals [142]. Now, several PDE4B and PDE4D selective inhibitors have been designed and synthesized, and their effects on inflammation are under investigation.

In summary: Managing psoriasis

Currently, there is no universal standard of care for patients with moderate to severe psoriasis, and the benefits and risks of systemic therapy must be weighed carefully for each patient to ensure optimal management of psoriasis symptoms and minimization of acute and cumulative toxicities [143]. Whether the symptoms are mild, moderate, or severe, the optimal treatment plan is the one the patient is most likely to follow. For those with localized disease, topical therapy is a suitable first choice. Phototherapy is generally the first-line treatment for patients with extensive psoriasis or disabling symptoms. When phototherapy is not feasible or is ineffective, systemic treatments with conventional oral agents or biologics are indicated [144]. Psoriasis is a common skin disorder that needs long-term management, not only because of its prevalence but also because of the profound impact it can have on quality of life.

Author details

F.Z. Zangeneh* and F.S. Shooshtary

*Address all correspondence to: Zangeneh14@gmail.com

Farideh Zafari Zangeneh, Vali-e-Asr, Reproductive Health Research Center, Imam Khomaini Hospital, Tehran University of Medical Sciences, Tehran, Iran

References

[1] Willan R.On Cutaneous Diseases. London: Johnson; 1808.

[2] Nestle FO, Kaplan DH, Barker J. Psoriasis. N. Engl. J. Med. 2009; 361: 496–509.

[3] Lebwohl M, Menter A, Koo J, Feldman S.Case studies in severe psoriasis: A clinical strategy. J Dermatolog Treat. 2003; 14 Suppl 2: 26-46.

[4] Naldi L, Mercuri SR. Smoking and psoriasis: from epidemiology to pathomechanisms. J Invest Dermatol. 2009; 129: 2741-3.

[5] Silman AJ, Hochberg MC. Psoriatic arthropathy. Epidemiology of the rheumatic diseases, Oxford University Press, New York (1993), pp. 86–104.

[6] aNaldi L. Epidemiology of psoriasis. Curr Drug Targets Inflamm Allergy. 2004; 3:121–128.

[7] aGriffiths CE, Barker JN. Pathogenesis and clinical features of psoriasis. Lancet. 2007; 370 (9583): 263-71.

[8] bGriffiths CE, Christophers E, Barker JN, Chalmers RJ, Chimenti S, Krueger GG, Leonardi C, Menter A, Ortonne JP, Fry L. A classification of psoriasis vulgaris according to phenotype. Br J Dermatol. 2007; 156: 258-62.

[9] Henseler T, Christophers E. Psoriasis of early and late onset: characterization of two types of psoriasis vulgaris. J Am Acad Dermatol 1985; 13:450–6.

[10] Goodfield M, Hull SM, Holland D, Roberts G, Wood E, Reid S, Cunliffe W. Investigations of the 'active' edge of plaque psoriasis: vascular proliferation precedes changes in epidermal keratin. Br J Dermatol 1994; 131: 808–13.

[11] bNaldi L, Colombo P, Benedetti EP, Piccitto R, Chatenoud L, La Vecchia C. Study design and preliminary results from the pilot phase of the PraKtis study: self-reported

diagnoses of selected skin diseases in a representative sample of the Italian population. Dermatology. 2004; 208: 38–42.

[12] Beylot C. Clinical aspects of psoriasis. Rev Prat 2004; 54: 19–27.

[13] Melski JW, Bernhard JD, Stern RS. The Koebner (isomorphic) response in psoriasis: associations with early age of onset and multiple previous therapies. Arch Dermatol. 1983; 119: 655–659.

[14] Zanchi M, Favot F, Bizzarini M, Piai M, Donini M, Sedona P. Botulinum toxin type-A for the treatment of inverse psoriasis. J Eur Acad Dermatol Venereol. 2008; 22: 431-6.

[15] Asumalahti K, Ameen, Suomela S, Hagforsen E, Michaëlsson G, Evans J, Munro M, Veal C, Allen M, Leman J, Burden AD, Kirby B, Connolly M, Griffiths CEM,Trembath RC, Kere G, Kere SU, Barker J NWN. Genetic analysis of PSORS1 distinguishes guttate psoriasis and palmoplantar pustulosis. J Invest Dermatol. 2003; 120: 627–632.

[16] Telfer NR, Chalmers RJ, Whale K, Colman G. The role of streptococcal infection in the initiation of guttate psoriasis. Arch Dermatol. 1992; 128: 39-42.

[17] Naldi L, Peli L, Parazzini F, Carrel CF. Family history of psoriasis, stressful life events, and recent infectious disease are risk factors for a first episode of acute guttate psoriasis: results of a case-control study. J Am Acad Dermatol. 2001; 44: 433–438.

[18] Mallon E, Bunce M, Savoie H, Rowe A, Newson R, Gotch F, Bunker CB. HLA-C and guttate psoriasis. Br J Dermatol. 2000; 143: 1177-82.

[19] Loh (No authors listed, Dr. Loh Correspondence): Acute Guttate Psoriasis in a 15-Year-Old Girl With Epstein-Barr Virus infection. Arch Dermatol. 2012; 148: 658-659.

[20] Zelickson BD, Muller SA. Generalised pustular psoriasis. A review of 63 cases. Arch Dermatol. 1991; 127: 1339–1345.

[21] Viguier M, Allez M, ZagdanskiAM High frequency of cholestasis in generalised pustular psoriasis. Evidence for neutrophilic involvement of the biliary tract. Hepatology. 2004; 40: 452–458.

[22] Sidoroff A, Halevy S, Bavinck JN, Vaillant L, Roujeau JC. Acute generalized exanthematous pustulosis (AGEP) a clinical reaction pattern. J Cutan Pathol. 2001; 28: 113–119.

[23] Saissi EH, Beau-Salinas F, Jonville-Bera AP, Lorette G, Autret-Leca E. Drugs associated with acute generalized exanthematic pustulosis. Ann Dermatol Venereol. 2003; 130: 612–618.

[24] Roelandts R. The history of phototherapy: something new under the sun? J Am Acad Dermatol. 2002; 46: 926-30.

[25] O'Doherty CJ, MacIntyre C. Palmoplantar pustulosis and smoking. 1985; 291: 861–864.

[26] Balasubramaniam P, Berth-Jones J. Erythroderma: 90% skin failure. Hosp Med. 2004; 65: 100–102.

[27] Kahl C, Hansen B, Reich K. Nail psoriasis--an ignored disorder. Pathogenesis, diagnosis and therapy. Hautarzt. 2012; 63: 184-91.

[28] Salomon J, Szepietowski JC, Proniewicz A. Psoriatic nails: a prospective clinical study. J Cutan Med Surg. 2003; 7: 317–321.

[29] Gelfand JM, Gladman DD, Mease PJ, Smith N, Margolis DJ, Nijsten T, Stern RS, Feldman SR, Rolstad T. Epidemiology of psoriatic arthritis in the population of the United States. J Am Acad Dermatol. 2005; 53: 573.

[30] Wilson FC, Icen M, Crowson CS, McEvoy MT, Gabriel SE, Kremers HM. Incidence and clinical predictors of psoriatic arthritis in patients with psoriasis: a population-based study. Arthritis Rheum. 2009; 6: 233–239.

[31] Gaydukova I, Rebrov A, Nikitina N, Poddubnyy D. Decreased heart rate variability in patients with psoriatic arthritis. Clin Rheumatol. 2012 Jun 7. (Epub ahead of print)

[32] Kane D, Stafford L, Bresnihan B, FitzGerald O. A prospective, clinical and radiological study of early psoriatic arthritis: an early synovitis clinic experience. Rheumatology (Oxford). 2003; 42: 1460-8.

[33] Baran R. The burden of nail psoriasis: an introduction. Dermatology. 2010; 221 Suppl 1:1-5.

[34] Takayanagi H. Osteoimmunology and the effects of the immune system on bone. Nat Rev Rheumatol. 2009; 5: 667-76.

[35] Rahimi H, Ritchlin CT. Altered bone biology in psoriatic arthritis. Curr Rheumatol Rep. 2012; 14: 349-57.

[36] Tada T. The immune system as a supersystem. Annu Rev Immunol. 1997; 15:1–13.

[37] Elenkov IJ, Webster EL, Torpy DJ, Chrousos GP. Stress, corticotropin-releasing hormone, glucocorticoids, and the immune/inflammatory response: acute and chronic effects. Ann NY Acad Sci. 1999; 876; 1– 11 (discussion 11-3).

[38] Grubauer G, Feingold KR, Elias PM.Relationship of epidermal lipogenesis to cutaneous barrier function. J Lipid Res. 1987 ; 28: 746-52.

[39] Stark HJ, Boehnke K, Mirancea N, Willhauck MJ, Pavesio A, Fusenig NE, Boukamp P.Epidermal homeostasis in long-term scaffold-enforced skin equivalents. J Investig Dermatol Symp Proc. 2006; 11: 93-105.

[40] Blanpain, C. Fuchs, E. Epidermal homeostasis: a balancing act of stem cells in the skin. Molecular Cell Biology. 2009; 10, 207-217.

[41] Ovaere P, Lippens S, Vandenabeele P, Declercq W. The emerging roles of serine protease cascades in the epidermis. Trends in Biochemical Sciences. 2009; 34: 453–463.

[42] Candi E, Schmidt R, Melino G. The cornified envelope: a model of cell death in the skin Nat. Rev. Mol. Cell Biol. 2005; 6: 328–340.

[43] Hannun, YA. Obeid, LM. Principles of bioactive lipid signaling: lessons from sphingolipids. Nature Reviews: Molecular Cell Biology. 2008; 9: 139–150.

[44] Harding CR, Watkinson A, Rawlings AV et al. Dry skin, moisturization and corneodesmolysis. Int J Cosmet Sci 2000; 22: 21–52.

[45] Ya-Xian Z., Suetake T., Tagami H. Number of cell layers of the stratum corneum in normal skin—relationship to the anatomical location on the body, age, sex and physical parameters. Arch Dermatol Res. 1999; 291: 555–9.

[46] Madison K C. Barrier function of the skin: "la raison d'etre" of the epidermis. J Invest Dermatol 2003: 121: 231–242.

[47] Caubet C, Jonca N, Brattsand M, Guerrin M, Bernard D, Schmidt R, Egelrud T, Simon M, Serre G. Degradation of corneodesmosome proteins by two serine proteases of the kallikrein family, SCTE/KLK5/hK5 and SCCE/KLK7/hK7. J Invest Dermatol. 2004; 122: 1235-44.

[48] Brattsand M, Egelrud T. Purification, molecular cloning, and expression of a human stratum corneum trypsin-like serine protease with possible function in desquamation. J Biol Chem. 1999; 274: 30033-40.

[49] Ekholm IE, Brattsand M, Egelrud T. Stratum corneum tryptic enzyme in normal epidermis: a missing link in the desquamation process? J Invest Dermatol. 2000; 114: 56–63.

[50] Meyer-Hoffert U.Reddish, scaly, and itchy: how proteases and their inhibitors contribute to inflammatory skin diseases. Arch Immunol Ther Exp (Warsz). 2009; 57: 345-54.

[51] Hachem JP, Wagberg F, Schmuth M, Crumrine D, Lissens W, Jayakumar A, Houben E, Mauro TM, Leonardsson G, Brattsand M, Egelrud T, Roseeuw D, Clayman GL, Feingold KR, Williams ML, Elias PM. Serine protease signaling of epidermal permeability barrier homeostasis. J Invest Dermatol. 2006; 126: 2074–2086.

[52] Kanitakis J. Anatomy, histology and immunohistochemistry of normal human skin. European Journal of Dermatology. 2002; 12: 390-401.

[53] Hennings H, Michael D, Cheng C, Steinert P, Holbrook K, Yuspa SH. Calcium regulation of growth and differentiation of mouse epidermal cells in culture. Cell. 1980; 19: 245-54.

[54] Schallreuter KU, Wood JM, Pittelkow MR, Swanson NN, Steinkraus V. Increased in vitro expression of beta 2-adrenoceptors in differentiating lesional keratinocytes of vitiligo patients. Arch Dermatol Res. 1993; 285: 216-20.

[55] Tausk F, Christian E, Johansson O, Milgram S. Neurobiology of the skin. T. B. Fitzpatrick, and A. Z. Eisen, and K. Wolff, and I. M. Freedberg, and K. F. Austen, eds. Dermatology in General Medicine 1993, 396 McGraw-Hill, New York.

[56] Tseraidis GS, Bavykina E A. Adrenergic innervation of normal human skin Vestn. Dermatol. Venerol.1972; 45: 40-45.

[57] Pullar, C. E., Isseroff, R. R and Nuccitelli, R. Cyclic AMP-dependent protein kinase A plays a role in the directed migration of human keratinocytes in a DC electric field. Cell Motil. Cytoskeleton. 2001; 50: 207-217.

[58] Strigl, R. Pfeiffer, U. Aschenbrenner, G. Blumel, G. Influence of the beta-1 selective blocker, metoprolol, on the development of pulmonary edema in tocolytic therapy. Obstet Gynecol. 1986; 67: 537–544.

[59] Inagaki, N. Miura, T. Daikoku, M. Nagai, H. Koda, A. Inhibitory effects of beta-adrenergic stimulants on increased vascular permeability caused by passive cutaneous anaphylaxis, allergic mediators, and mediator releasers in rats. Pharmacolog.. 1989; 39: 19–27.

[60] Paul, W. Douglas, GJ. Lawrence, L. Khawaja, M. Perez, AC. Schacter M. Cutaneous permeability responses to bradykinin and histamine in the guinea-pig: possible differences in their mechanism of action. Br J Pharmacol. 1994; 111: 159–164.

[61] Ding, Z. Jiang, M. Li, S. Zhang,Y. Vascular barrier-enhancing effect of an endogenous beta-adrenergic agonist. Inflammation. 1995; 19: 1–8.

[62] Dyess, DL. Hunter, JL. Lakey, JR. Moyer, D. Dougherty, FC. Townsley, MI. Attenuation of histamine-induced endothelial permeability responses after pacing-induced heart failure: role for endogenous catecholamines. Microcirculation. 2000; 7: 307–315.

[63] Broadley KJ. Review of mechanisms involved in the apparent differential desensitization of beta1- and beta2-adrenoceptor-mediated functional responses. J Auton Pharmacol. 1999; 19: 335-45.

[64] Johnson M. Beta2-adrenoceptors: mechanisms of action of beta2-agonists. Paediatr Respir Rev. 2001; 2: 57-62.

[65] Spina D. "PDE4 inhibitors: current status". British Journal of Pharmacology. 2008; 155: 308–315.

[66] Eedy DJ, Canavan JP, Shaw C, Trimble ER. Beta-adrenergic stimulation of cyclic AMP is defective in cultured dermal fibroblasts of psoriatic subjects. Br. J. Dermatol. 1990; 122: 477-483.

[67] Gazith J, Cavey MT, Cavey D, Shroot B, Reichert U. Characterization of the beta-adrenergic receptors of cultured human epidermal keratinocytes. Biochem Pharmacol. 1983; 32: 3397-403.

[68] Schallreuter KU, Lemke KR, Pittelkow MR, Wood JM, Körner C & Malik R. Catecholamines in human keratinocyte differentiation. J Invest Dermatol. 1995; 104: 953–957.

[69] Koizumi H, Yasui C, Fukaya T, Ohkawara A, Ueda T. Beta-adrenergic stimulation induces intracellular Ca++ increase in human epidermal keratinocytes. J Invest Dermatol. 1991; 96: 234-7.

[70] Koizumi H, Tanaka H, Ohkawara A. beta-Adrenergic stimulation induces activation of protein kinase C and inositol 1,4,5-trisphosphate increase in epidermis. Exp Dermatol. 1997; 6(3): 128-32.

[71] Karvonen SL, Korkiamäki T, Ylä-Outinen H, Nissinen M, Teerikangas H, Pummi K, Karvonen J, Peltonen J. Psoriasis and altered calcium metabolism: downregulated capacitative calcium influx and defective calcium-mediated cell signaling in cultured psoriatic keratinocytes. J Invest Dermatol. 2000; 114: 693-700.

[72] Lebre MC, van der Aar AM, van Baarsen L, van Capel TM, Schuitemaker JH, Kapsenberg ML, de Jong EC.Human keratinocytes express functional Toll-like receptor 3, 4, 5, and 9. J Invest Dermatol. 2007; 127: 331-41.

[73] Wood, LC. Jackson, SM. Elias, PM. Grunfeld, C. Feingold, KR. Cutaneous barrier perturbation stimulates cytokine production in the epidermis of mice. J Clin Invest. 1992; 90: 482–487.

[74] Wood, LC. Stalder, AK. Liou, A. Barrier disruption increases gene expression of cytokines and the 55 kD TNF receptor in murine skin. Exp Dermatol. 1997; 6: 98–104.

[75] Jensen JM, Schütze S, Förl M, Krönke M, Proksch E. Roles for tumor necrosis factor receptor p55 and sphingomyelinase in repairing the cutaneous permeability barrier. J Clin Invest. 1999; 104: 1761-70.

[76] Wang XP, Schunck M, Kallen KJ, Neumann C, Trautwein C, Rose-John S, Proksch E. The interleukin-6 cytokine system regulates epidermal permeability barrier homeostasis. J Invest Dermatol. 2004; 123: 124-31.

[77] Hardardottir, I. Kunitake, St. Moser, AH. Endotoxin and cytokines increase hepatic messenger RNA levels and serum concentrations of apolipoprotein J (clusterin) in Syrian hamsters. J Clin Invest. 1994; 94: 1304–1309.

[78] Barland, CO. Zettersten, E. Brown, BS. Ye, J. Elias, PM. Ghadially, R. Imiquimod-induced interleukin-1 alpha stimulation improves barrier homeostasis in aged murine epidermis. J Invest Dermatol. 2004; 122: 330–336.

[79] Besedovsky, H. O., Del Rey, A. E., Sorkin, E. Immune-neuroendocrine interactions J. Immunol. 1985; 135: 750s-754s.

[80] Kin NW, Sanders VM. It takes nerve to tell T and B cells what to do. J Leukoc Biol. 2006; 79: 1093-104.

[81] Schallreuter KU. Epidermal adrenergic signal transduction as part of the neuronal network in the human epidermis. J. Investig. Dermatol. Symp. Proc 1997; 2: 37–40.

[82] Ionescu G, Kiehl R. Increased plasma norepinephrine in psoriasis. Acta Derm Venereol. 1991; 71: 169-170.

[83] Schmid-Ott G, Jacobs R, Jäger B, Klages S, Wolf J, Werfel T, Kapp A, Schürmeyer T, Lamprecht F, Schmidt RE, Schedlowski M. Stress-induced endocrine and immunological changes in psoriasis patients and healthy controls. A preliminary study. Psychother Psychosom. 1998; 67: 37-42.

[84] Zangeneh FZ, Fazeli A.The significance of stress hormones in Psoriasis. Acta Medica Iranica. 2008; 46: 485-488.

[85] Johansson O, Olsson A, Enhamre A, Hammar H, Goldstein M. Phenylethanolamine N-methyltransferase-like immunoreactivity in psoriasis. An immunohistochemical study on catecholamine synthesizing enzymes and neuropeptides of the skin. Acta Derm Venereol. 1987; 67: 1-7.

[86] Padgett DA, Glaser R. How stress influences the immune response. Trends Immunol. 2003; 24: 444–448.

[87] Halevy S, Livni E. Beta-adrenergic blocking drugs and psoriasis: the role of an immunologic mechanism. J. Am. Acad. Dermatol. 1993; 29: 504–505.

[88] Yilmaz MB, Turhan H, Akin Y, Kisacik HL, Korkmaz S. Beta-blocker-induced psoriasis: a rare side effect—a case report. Angiology. 2002; 53: 737–739.

[89] Gisondi P, Ferrazzi A, Girolomoni G.Metabolic comorbidities and psoriasis. Acta Dermatovenerol Croat. 2010;18: 297-304.

[90] Bergboer JG, Zeeuwen PL, Schalkwijk J.Genetics of Psoriasis: Evidence for Epistatic Interaction between Skin Barrier Abnormalities and Immune Deviation. J Invest Dermatol. 2012 May 24. doi: 10.1038/jid.2012.167. (Epub ahead of print)

[91] Wu JJ, Nguyen TU, Poon KY, Herrinton LJ.The association of psoriasis with autoimmune diseases. J Am Acad Dermatol. 2012 Jun 2. (Epub ahead of print)

[92] Bonnet MC, Preukschat D, Welz PS, van Loo G, Ermolaeva MA, Bloch W, Haase I, Pasparakis M.The adaptor protein FADD protects epidermal keratinocytes from necroptosis in vivo and prevents skin inflammation. Immunity. 2011; 35: 572-82.

[93] Nance DM, Sanders VM. Autonomic innervation and regulation of the immune system. Brain Behav Immun. 2007; 21: 736-45.

[94] Kleyn CE, McKie S, Ross AR, Montaldi D, Gregory LJ, Elliott R, Isaacs CL, Anderson IM, Richards HL, Deakin JF, Fortune DG, Griffiths CE. Diminished neural and cognitive responses to facial expressions of disgust in patients with psoriasis: a functional magnetic resonance imaging study. J Invest Dermatol. 2009; 129: 2613-9.

[95] Gisondi P, Girolomoni G, Sampogna F, Tabolli S, Abeni D. Prevalence of psoriatic arthritis and joint complaints in a large population of Italian patients hospitalized for psoriasis. Eur J Dermatol. 2005; 15:279–83.

[96] Kimball AB, Jacobson C, Weiss S, Vreeland MG, Wu Y. The psychosocial burden of psoriasis. Am J Clin Dermatol 2005; 6:383–92.

[97] Henseler T, Christophers E. Disease concomitance in psoriasis. J Am Acad Dermatol 1995; 32:982–6.

[98] Mallbris L, Ritchlin CT, Ståhle M. Metabolic disorders in patients with psoriasis and psoriatic arthritis. Current Rheumatology Reports, 2006; 8: 355–363.

[99] Gelfand JM, Neimann AL, Shin DB et al. Risk of myocardial infarction in patients with psoriasis. JAMA. 2006; 296:1735–41.

[100] Ziegler MG, Elayan H, Milic M, Sun P, Gharaibeh M. Epinephrine and the metabolic syndrome. Curr Hypertens Rep. 2012; 14: 1-7.

[101] Gelfand JM, Yeung H. Metabolic syndrome in patients with psoriatic disease. J Rheumatol Suppl. 2012; 89: 24-8.

[102] Neimann et al. "Prevalence of Cardiovascular Risk Factors in Patients with Psoriasis." J Am Acad Dermatol. 2006; 55: 829-35.

[103] Mehta NN, Azfar RS, Shin DB, Neimann AL, Troxel AB, Gelfand JM.Patients with severe psoriasis are at increased risk of cardiovascular mortality: cohort study using the General Practice Research Database. Eur Heart J. 2010; 31: 1000-6.

[104] aAugustin M, Reich K, Glaeske G, Schaefer I, Radtke M. Co-morbidity and age-related prevalence of psoriasis: analysis of health insurance data in Germany. Acta Derm Venereol 2010; 90: 147–151.

[105] bAugustin M, Glaeske G, Radtke MA, Christophers E, Reich K, Schafer I. Epidemiology and comorbidity of psoriasis in children. Br J Dermatol 2010; 162: 633–636.

[106] Denda M, Fuziwara S, Inoue K. ß2-Adrenergic Receptor Antagonist Accelerates Skin Barrier Recovery and Reduces Epidermal Hyperplasia Induced by Barrier Disruption. Journal of Investigative Dermatology. 2003; 121: 142–148.

[107] aTakahashi H, Kinouchi M, Tamura T, Iizuka H. Decreased beta 2-adrenergic receptor-mRNA and loricrin-mRNA, and increased involucrin-mRNA transcripts in psoriatic epidermis: analysis by reverse transcription-polymerase chain reaction. Br J Dermatol. 1996; 134: 1065-9.

[108] Freund YR, Akama T, Alley MR, Antunes J, Dong C, Jarnagin K, Kimura R, Nieman JA, Maples KR, Plattner JJ, Rock F, Sharma R, Singh R, Sanders V, Zhou Y. Boron-based phosphodiesterase inhibitors show novel binding of boron to PDE4 bimetal center. FEBS Lett. 2012 Jul 25. [Epub ahead of print]

[109] bTakahashi H, Tamura T, Iizuka H. 1,25-Dihydroxyvitamin D3 increased beta-adrenergic adenylate cyclase response of fetal rat keratinizing epidermal cells (FRSK cells) J Dermatol Sci. 1996;11: 121–128.

[110] Takahashi H, Iizuka H. Regulation of beta 2-adrenergic receptors in keratinocytes: glucocorticoids increase steady-state levels of receptor mRNA in foetal rat keratinizing epidermal cells (FRSK cells). Br J Dermatol. 1991; 124: 341-7.

[111] Iizuka H, Kajita S, Ohkawara A. Ultraviolet radiation augments epidermal beta-adrenergic adenylate cyclase response. J Invest Dermatol. 1985; 84: 401–403.

[112] Cather J, Menter A. Novel therapies for psoriasis. Am J Clin Dermatol 2002; 3: 159–173.

[113] Nast A, Kopp I, Augustin M et al. German evidence-based guidelines for the treatment of Psoriasis vulgaris (short version). Arch Dermatol Res 2007; 299: 111–138.

[114] Menter A, Korman NJ, Elmets CA et al. Guidelines of care for the management of psoriasis and psoriatic arthritis. Section 3. Guidelines of care for the management and treatment of psoriasis with topical therapies. J Am Acad Dermatol 2009; 60: 643–659.

[115] Murphy G, Reich K. In touch with psoriasis: topical treatments and current guidelines. J Eur Acad Dermatol Venereol 2011; 25: 3–8.

[116] Mason AR, Mason J, Cork M, Dooley G, Edwards G. Topical treatments for chronic plaque psoriasis. Cochrane Database Syst Rev. 2009; 15: CD005028.

[117] Juzeniene A, Moan J. Beneficial effects of UV radiation other than via vitamin D production. Dermatoendocrinol. 2012; 4: 109-17.

[118] Walker D, Jacobe H. Phototherapy in the age of biologics. Semin Cutan Med Surg. 2011; 30: 190-8.

[119] Bulat V, Situm M, Dediol I, Ljubicić I, Bradić L. The mechanisms of action of phototherapy in the treatment of the most common dermatoses. Coll Antropol. 2011; 35:147-51.

[120] Pavel S. Light therapy (with UVA-1) for SLE patients: is it a good or bad idea? Rheumatology (Oxford). 2006; 45: 653-5.

[121] Mang R, Krutmann J. UVA-1 Phototherapy. Photodermatol Photoimmunol Photomed. 2005; 21: 103-8.

[122] Xiang Y, Liu G, Yang L, Zhong JL. UVA-induced protection of skin through the induction of heme oxygenase-1. Biosci Trends. 2011; 5: 239-44.

[123] Roelandts R. The history of phototherapy: something new under the sun? J Am Acad Dermatol. 2002; 46: 926-30.

[124] Gottlieb AB. Psoriasis. Dis Manag Clin Outcomes 1998; 1: 195–202.

[125] Tristani-Firouzi P, Krueger GG. Efficacy and safety of treatment modalities for psoriasis. Cutis 1998; 61 (Suppl.): 11–21.

[126] Griffiths CEM, Clark CM, Chalmers RJG et al. A systematic review of treatments for severe psoriasis. Health Technol Assess 2000; 4: 1–125.

[127] Lebwohl M, Drake L, Menter A et al. Consensus conference: acitretin in combination with UVB or PUVA in the treatment of psoriasis. J Am Acad Dermatol 2001; 45: 544–53.

[128] Tolman KG, Clegg DD, Lee RG, Ward JR. Methotrexate and liver. J Rheumatol Suppl 1985; 12: 29–34.

[129] Kumar B, Saraswat A, Kaur I. Short-term methotrexate therapy in psoriasis: a study of 197 patients. Int J Dermatol 2002; 41: 444–448.

[130] Mueller W, Herrmann B. Cyclosporin A for psoriasis. N Engl J Med 1979; 301: 555.

[131] Treumer F, Zhu K, Glaser R et al. Dimethylfumarate is a potent inducer of apoptosis in human T cells. J Invest Dermatol 2003; 121: 1383–8.

[132] Mrowietz U, Christophers E, Altmeyer P. Treatment of severe psoriasis with fumaric acid esters: scientific background and guidelines for therapeutic use. The German Fumaric Acid Ester Consensus Conference. Br J Dermatol 1999; 141: 424–9.

[133] Tobin AM, Kirby B. TNF alpha inhibitors in the treatment of psoriasis and psoriatic arthritis. BioDrugs. 2005; 19: 47-57.

[134] Wendling D, Balblanc JC, Briançon D, Brousse A, Lohse A, Deprez P, Humbert P, Aubin F. Onset or exacerbation of cutaneous psoriasis during TNFalpha antagonist therapy. Joint Bone Spine. 2008; 75: 315-8.

[135] Puig L, Morales-Múnera CE, López-Ferrer A, Geli C. Ustekinumab Treatment of TNF Antagonist-Induced Paradoxical Psoriasis Flare in a Patient with Psoriatic Arthritis: Case Report and Review. Dermatology. 2012 Aug 10. (Epub ahead of print).

[136] Torphy TJ. Phosphodiesterase isozymes: molecular targets for novel antiasthma agents. Am J Respir Crit Care Med. 1998; 157: 351-70.

[137] Houslay MD, Schafer P, Zhang KY. Keynote review: phosphodiesterase-4 as a therapeutic target. Drug Discov Today. 2005; 10: 1503-19.

[138] Jin SLC, Richter W, Conti M. Insights into the physiological functions of PDE4 from knockout mice. In: Beavo JA, Francis SH, Houslay MD, eds. Cyclic Nucleotide Phosphodiesterases in Health and Disease Boca Raton, FL: CRC Press. 2007:323-46.

[139] Naganuma K, Omura A, Maekawara N, Saitoh M, Ohkawa N, Kubota T, Nagumo H, Kodama T, Takemura M, Ohtsuka Y, Nakamura J, Tsujita R, Kawasaki K, Yokoi H, Kawanishi M. Discovery of selective PDE4B inhibitors. Bioorg Med Chem Lett 2009; 19: 3174-6.

[140] Nazarian R, Weinberg JM. AN-2728, a PDE4 inhibitor for the potential topical treatment of psoriasis and atopic dermatitis. Curr Opin Investig Drugs. 2009; 10: 1236-42.

[141] Higgs G. Is PDE4 too difficult a drug target? Curr Opin Investig Drugs. 2010; 11: 495-8.

[142] McCann FE, Palfreeman AC, Andrews M, Perocheau DP, Inglis JJ, Schafer P, Feldmann M, Williams RO, Brennan FM. Apremilast, a novel PDE4 inhibitor, inhibits spontaneous production of tumour necrosis factor-alpha from human rheumatoid synovial cells and ameliorates experimental arthritis. Arthritis Res Ther. 2010; 12: R107.

[143] Naldi L, Griffiths CE. Traditional therapies in the management of moderate to severe chronic plaque psoriasis: an assessment of the benefits and risks. Br J Dermatol. 2005; 152: 597-615.

[144] Uhlenhake EE, Mehregan DA. Managing psoriasis: what's best for your patient? J Fam Pract. 2012; 61: 402-9, 451.

Chapter 2

Clinical Presentation of Psoriasis

Ananya Datta Mitra and Anupam Mitra

Additional information is available at the end of the chapter

http://dx.doi.org/10.5772/55866

1. Introduction

Psoriasis, a chronic papulosquamous inflammatory skin disease, was originally thought of as a primary disorder of epidermal keratinocytes, but is later on recognized as one of the commonest immune-mediated disorders [1, 2]. Although psoriasis starts with the involvement of skin, but limiting this disease to a skin problem is rather a restrictive approach. Psoriasis has been linked to a number of other diseases especially metabolic derangements and arthritis [3-5]. The disease imparts a huge socio-economic burden [6, 7] and the diagnosis of psoriasis is purely based on clinical features. Depending upon the type of psoriasis, onset may be abrupt or slowly progressive. Although it may appear at any age, but majority of patients experience the first episode before the age of 40 years and is uncommon before 10 years [8]. The population based study at Mayo Clinic, suggest that psoriasis tends to appear at an earlier age in females compared to males [9]. A study by Henseler et al. suggested that many psoriatic patients show bimodal distribution i.e. peak between 16-22 years and later between 57-60 years [2, 10].

2. Epidemiology of psoriasis

Psoriasis shows a worldwide prevalence. The estimate of prevalence psoriasis varies among different ethnic groups and also by geographical location, more common in colder northern zone compared to tropical zone and has been reported to vary in between 0 to 11.8% [11, 12]. Several confounding factors need to be taken into consideration for analyzing the prevalence data of psoriasis namely: method of ascertainment (population based, clinic based, questionnaire based), age and type of prevalence estimated (point, period, lifetime) [8, 13]. Taking into consideration of the confounding factors, the prevalence of psoriasis is highest in northern Europeans and almost absent in aboriginal population of south America [11]. In United States, the prevalence of psoriasis ranges between 2.2% to 2.6% and is lower in African-american compared to Caucasians. The prevalence rate of psoriasis in China and Japan is low than European ethnicity and in India it ranges between 0.5% to 2.3% [8, 13-15].

3. Latent, minimal and overt psoriasis

The course of the disease in the same individual is not uniform over time. It may range from apparently healthy to minor signs to overt clinical manifestations. No diagnostic test is available to predict future psoriasis development, that's why the diagnosis of "latent psoriasis" in individuals without a previous history of the disease remains impossible. On the other hand, the diagnosis of "minimal psoriasis" largely depends on subjective variation due to lack of validated criteria. The minor signs of psoriasis, which are also known as 'stigmata of psoriasis' are described in Table 1, but their contribution to overt psoriasis remains unknown.

Hyperkeratotic plaques on the exterior surface without scaling
Keratolysis like lesions of the palms and soles
Eczematous patches on palms and soles
Severe dandruff
Nail pitting
Sterile multiple paronychia
Subungual hyperkeratosis and onycholysis without fungal infection
Recalcitrant scaly otitis externa
Intertrigo with sharp marginated erythema
Sharply marginated penile erythema without fungal infection

Table 1. Stigmata of psoriasis [16]

4. Classifying psoriasis: The clinical spectrum

Psoriasis is a disease of coexisting signs and symptoms characterized by scaly, erythematous lesions with sharply demarcated margins. It's interesting to note that scaling prevails in the stable chronic plaque stage of psoriasis and erythema predominates in the unstable progressing lesions of guttate psoriasis. The lesions are itchy and bleed easily. One of the classical sign of psoriasis is the 'Auspitz' sign, characterized by pinpoint bleeding when outer scales are removed from psoriatic plaques. Psoriasis cannot be classified based on a single factor and generally involves differentiation of lesions based on: a. morphology of the lesions, b. degree of inflammation, c. distributing patterns of the lesions, d. extent of body surface involvement, e. first onset and f. velocity of propagation [17].

http://dx.doi.org/10.5772/55866

4.1. Chronic plaque psoriasis

This is the commonest form of psoriasis, represents 70-80% of psoriatic patients and is also known as Psoriasis vulgaris. The patient presented with sharply demarcated round-oval, or nummular (coin-sized) plaques with a loosely adherent silvery white scale, specially affecting the elbows, knees, lumbosacral areal, intergluteal cleft and scalp (Figure 1 & 2). The lesions usually begin as erythematous macules or papules, extend peripherally, and coalesce to form plaques. Woronoff's ring, a white blanching ring may be observed in the skin surrounding a psoriatic plaque [18, 19]. The gradual peripheral extension of the plaques resulting in different configurations including:

a. psoriasis gyrate: predominantly curved linear pattern

b. annular psoriasis: ring like lesions develop secondary to central clearing

c. psoriasis follicularis: presence of tiny scaly papules at the openings of pilosebaceous follicles

Occasionally, presence of lesions on the scalp and face makes it difficult to separate this variety from seborrheic dermatitis (sebopsoriasis). There are two distinct morphological subtypes of plaque psoriasis: Rupioid and Ostraceous. Rupioid plaques resembles limpet shells, small (2-5 cm in diameter) and highly hyperkeratotic. Ostraceous psoriasis is characterized by hyper-keratotic plaques, relatively concave centres, resembles oyster shells. Scale is typically present in psoriasis, is characteristically silvery white, and can vary in thickness. Removal of scale may reveal tiny bleeding points (Auspitz sign). The amount of scaling varies among patients and even at different sites on a given patient. Apart from its usual presentation, chronic plaque psoriasis sometimes affecting the flexures such as inframammary, axillary and perineal region known as *inverse psoriasis.* Inverse psoriatic lesions have minimal or no scales and appear as red, shiny, well demarcated plaques and may be confused with candidal, intertrigo, and dermatophyte infections.

The lesions are steady over time and as they regress, they start with central clearing with a peripheral activity margin which produces an annular or polycyclic appearance of the lesions. Central clearing is sometimes associated with hypopigmentation. Although the lesions are benign but may be complicated by appearance of inflammation with pustules and peripheral extension of the lesions.

4.2. Guttate psoriasis

Guttate psoriasis came from the Greek word 'gutta', which means droplet. Guttate psoriasis accounts for 2% of the total psoriasis [19]. This variety is distinguished by its acute onset of round erythematous exanthem (2-10 mm diameter) over the trunk and extremities in a centripetal fashion. The number of lesions may vary from 5 to more than 100 (Figure 3). Although the disease has a self limiting course, but a certain percentage of individuals may evolve to chronic plaque psoriasis. It is often reported that about 10% of psoriatic patients with the chronic plaque psoriasis have flares of guttate lesions during the course of their disease [18]. Guttate psoriasis commonly affect children or young adults with family history of

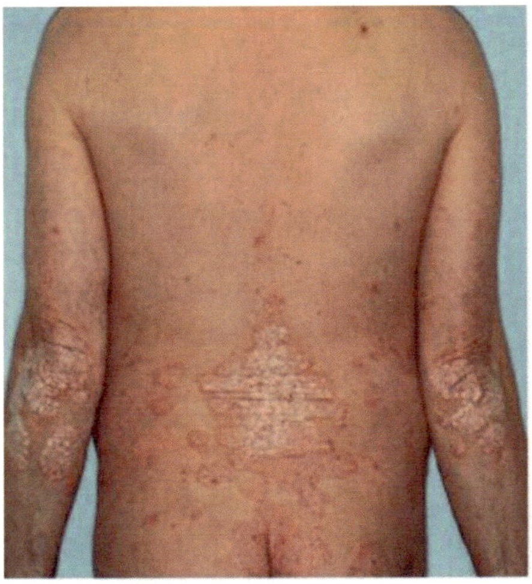

Figure 1. Localized plaque psoriasis

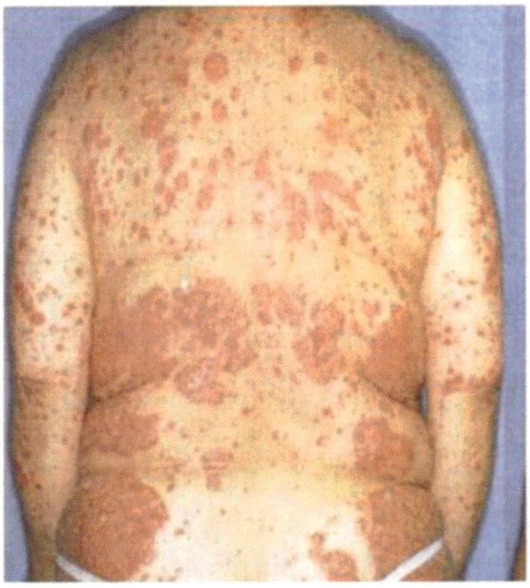

Figure 2. Generalized plaque psoriasis

psoriasis and may follow streptococcal infection and/or acute stressful life events [20]. It is estimated that there is a 40% increased risk of developing chronic psoriasis after a bout of guttate variety [21]. It's quite interesting to note that chronic plaque psoriasis and guttate psoriasis appear to be genetically similar with a strong association to the *PSORS1* genetic locus, which is also a major determinant of Psoriasis vulgaris [22, 23].

4.3. Generalized pustular psoriasis (von Zumbusch)

Generalized pustular psoriasis is rare and represents active, unstable disease. Population survey reports that almost 20% of patients have pustular lesions superimposed on lesions of

http://dx.doi.org/10.5772/55866

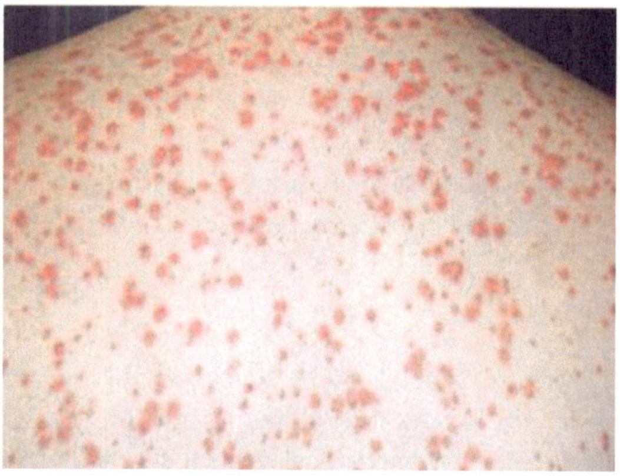

Figure 3. Guttate psoriasis

chronic plaque psoriasis at any time during the course of the disease [16]. However, only 2-5% of psoriatic patients have predominant pustular variety, having only pustules dominating the clinical picture [24]. Acute generalized pustular psoriasis generally develops after an irritant topical treatment of plaque psoriasis or due to abrupt corticosteroid withdrawal [25, 26]. Onset of an acute generalized pustular psoriasis is characterized by red and tender skin with systemic symptoms like fever, anorexia and nausea. Within hours, innumerable pustules appear with an erythematous background. Later on pustules become confluent creating ponds of pus with severe systemic symptoms. Consequently, the pustules dry and skin exfoliates producing a glazed erythematous surface where new crops of pustules might appear. There may be geographic tongue, polyarthritis and cholestasis associated with generalized pustular psoriasis [27]. Patients with generalized pustular psoriasis often need hospitalization for management. With remission of acute episodes, patient either follows an erythrodermic state or may produce plaque like lesions. Rarely, pustular psoriasis may appear during first six months of pregnancy, being called *impetigo herpetiformis* [28].

4.4. Localized pustular psoriasis

Localized pustular psoriasis includes two clinicaly distinct varieties: acrodermatitis continua of Hallopeau and palmoplantar pustulosis.

Acrodermatitis continua (dermatitis repens): A rare pustular eruption of the fingers and toes initiated after a localized trauma starting at the tip of a single digit [29]. Subsequently, the pustules become confluent and may spread proximally to involve the dorsal aspects of the hands, forearms and feet. Eventually, patients may develop osteolysis of the distal phalanx and associated onychodystrophy and anonychia of the involved digits. Sometimes the pustules become generalized.

Palmoplantar pustulosis: The characterizing feature of this variety is hyperkeratosis and clusters of sterile, yellow pustules on a background of erythema and scaling, affecting the ventral aspect of palms and/or soles. The pustules are tender and form dark brown color with adherent scales or crust. It is frequently associated with psoriatic nail involvement. In almost 25% cases, it is associated with psoriasis vulgaris, but it is now believed that palmoplantar pustulosis may not be a form of psoriasis due to lack of genetic association with PSORS1 locus. Moreover, it is predominant in women and is strongly associated with smoking [23, 30]. This disease has been associated with pustulotic arthroosteitis involving the anterior chest wall, sacroiliitis, and peripheral synovitis [31, 32]. Palmoplantar pustulosis is also an element of SAPHO syndrome, characterized by synovitis, acne, pustulosis, hyperostosis, and osteitis [33].

4.5. Erythrodermic psoriasis

Psoriatic erythroderma is characterized by extensive involvement of the skin by active psoriasis and represents in one of the two forms (Figure 4). In one form, chronic plaque psoriasis gradually progress and involve extensive body surface. In the second form which is more serious, erythroderma is a manifestation of unstable psoriasis, which is precipitated by triggers such as infection, tar, drugs and withdrawal of corticosteroids. This unstable form of psoriasis is characterize by prominent erythema and loss of characteristic clinical features of psoriasis [34]. Erythroderma impairs the thermoregulatory capacity of the skin resulting in hypothermia, high output cardiac failure, and metabolic changes, which needs immediate inpatient care.

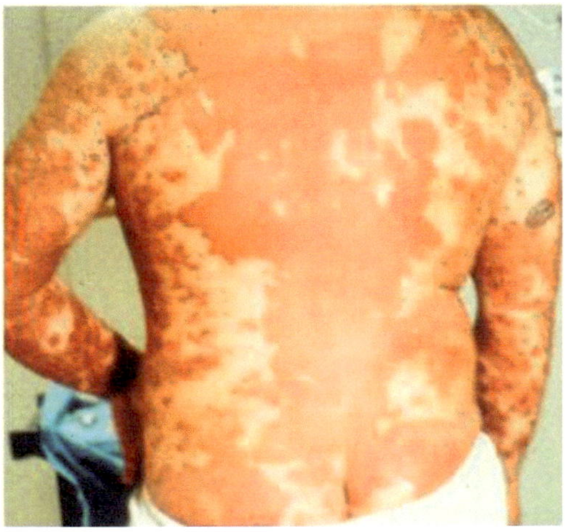

Figure 4. Erythrodermic psoriasis

4.6. Psoriatic nail disease

In psoriasis, finger nails are more commonly affected than toe nails. 'Pitting of nail' i.e. small pits in the nail plate are the commonest finding, resulting from defective nail formation in the proximal portion of the nail matrix. In addition, the nail may detach from the nail bed known as onycholysis and 'oil-spots' i.e. orange-yellow areas can be seen beneath the nail plate (Figure 5). Moreover, the nail plate may become, thickened, dystrophic, discolored and yellow, keratinous material may collect under the nail plate, which is known as subungual hyperker-

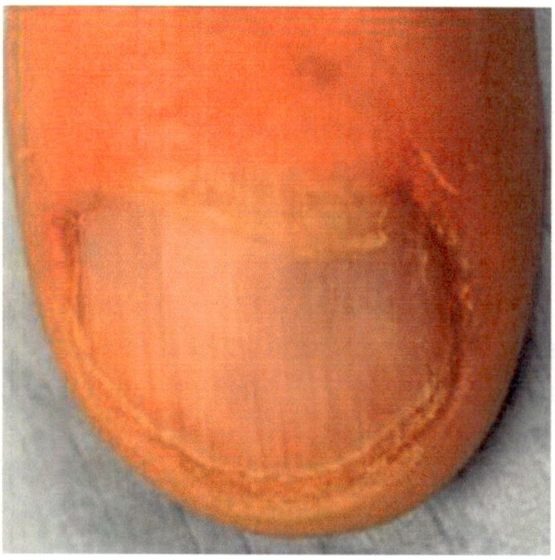

Figure 5. Nail changes

atosis. In most psoriatic patients, minor nail changes are observed and major nail abnormalities are usually associated with psoriatic arthritis and scalp involvement [19, 35].

5. Extension of the psoriatic spectrum beyond skin

Psoriasis is a systemic, chronic inflammatory disorder, occuring due to complex interplay of genetic, environmental and immunologic factors, predominantly affecting skin but can involve any organ systems of the body. Epidemiological studies in Caucasian and Asian populations show that patients with psoriasis suffer from other chronic inflammatory conditions with overlapping pathology, such as rheumatoid arthritis and inflammatory bowel disease, more frequently than patients without psoriasis [36, 37].

Psoriatic arthritis is a chronic inflammatory arthritis affecting about 5–25% of patients with psoriasis. The prevalence varies from 20–420 per 100,000 population across the world except in Japan where it is 1 per 100,000 [38]. Psoriatic arthritis has been defined as "an inflammatory arthritis occurring during the course of psoriasis and characterized by negative rheumatoid factor" [5]. Although arthritis typically occurs in fourth and fifth decade, no age is exempted with cases involving young children and elderly. There is no gender bias and both sexes are affected with a male to female ratio varying from 0.7:1 to 2.1:1. In majority of the patients (49–75%), arthritis follows chronic psoriasis of about 7–12 years duration. This follows onset of skin and joint disease in 10–37% patients simultaneously and lastly it can precede psoriasis in 6–18% [39-46]. Psoriatic arthritis is most commonly associated with psoriasis vulgaris. Conventionally, psoriatic arthritis can affect both the peripheral joints as well as the axial skeleton; thus, the joint involvement has been grouped into different subtypes. The original Moll and Wright classification criteria divided psoriatic arthritis into five subtypes: distal interphalangeal (DIP) predominant, symmetrical polyarthritis, single or few fingers or toe joints involved (asymmetrical oligoarthritis and monoarthritis), predominant spondylitis, and arthritis mutilans [47].

Psoriasis can be associated with a range of co-morbidities that include metabolic diseases, such as diabetes and cardiovascular (CV) diseases, tumors of specific sites, such as, lung cancer, colon cancer, and kidney cancer [48] and psychological disorders such as depression [49-55]. These comorbidities might influence patients' health and quality of life (QoL), and contribute to the 3 to 4 year reduction in life expectancy in patients of severe psoriasis [56]. There have been associations of psoriasis with smoking and increased body mass index [4, 57], which may influence clinical severity and prognosis. Established psoriasis has been associated with the several components of the metabolic syndrome, including hypertension, dyslipidemia, obesity, and impaired glucose tolerance [3, 49, 58]. It has been reported that suppression of the inflammatory process may reduce the cardiovascular risk in patients with psoriasis and rheumatoid arthritis [59, 60].

6. Grading the severity

Psoriasis, unlike many chronic disorders, does not emerge steadily toward a definite outcome, and therefore it is difficult to do staging of the disease by natural history [61]. Simple outcome measures like clinical remission, number of hospital admissions or ambulatory consultations and major disease flare-ups may affect disease severity. Measurement of disease severity only based on assessing skin area involvement at a point of time, has large limitations as it does not provide any direct information on the disease in terms of psychologic or social consequences. Moreover, differences between different pattern distributions or clinical subgroups in psoriasis except chronic plaque psoriasis, are inadequately addressed by these indices. The example for such measures is the Psoriasis Area and Severity Index (PASI), which was developed as an outcome measure in clinical trials on oral retinoids in 1978 [16, 62].

In this perspective, Quality of life (Qol) measures have the advantage of considering the multidimensional nature of disease assessment and outcome, which generally includes evaluation of disease related discomfort, level of disability and social disruption. However there is a limitation of their confirmation against a gold standard and the characterization of severity thresholds. Their use in clinical studies is still very limited. Qol refers to quantitative estimates acquired through standardized questionnaires exploring the relevant dimensions of the patient's life in terms of physical, social, and psychologic well being, that may be affected by the disease [63, 64]. Among the instruments designed for specifically assessing psoriasis are the Psoriasis Disability Index [65] and the Psoriasis Life Stress Inventory [66].

European Medicines Agency developed a set of criterion based on clinical features of psoriasis, involving a change in disease management from no treatment to topical and systemic modalities. These criterions are based on certain definitions which were developed to standardize assessment in randomized clinical trials. The definitions take into account; degree of skin involvement and patient's opinion as for example 1) Minimal disease with few isolated lesions and disease in remission with no psoriatic lesions, 2) Mild disease with PASI<10% and well controlled with topical treatment, 3) Moderate disease with PASI>10% and can be treated topically, 4) Moderate to severe disease with PASI>10% and failure of topical therapy or PASI<10% with disabling lesions in face, hands and feet, 4) Severe disease with PASI>20% or PASI>10% and <20% with disabling lesions in face, hands and feet and 5) Psoraisis with guarded prognosis including Generalized pustular psoriasis and psoriatic erythroderma [67]. A careful distinction between severe diseases versus disease affecting Qol severely has relevant implications in disease management. Studies report that patients with mild psoriasis having a severe impact on Qol can benefit from psychologic support than systemic drugs to suppress disease activity [62].

7. Disease prognosis

Due to its chronicity and incurability, psoriasis has a comparatively higher prevalence in the general population. Generally, with age, the point prevalence and the lifetime prevalence is anticipated to increase but in many studies it was shown that prevalence does not increase or even diminish with age [17]. This may be due to increased mortality among psoriatic patients later in life as compared to general population. Association with smoking and other comorbidities might contribute to such a drift [68]. It has also been reported that Qol indices might decline in long run independent of treatment [69]. Moreover, the progression of the skin lesions does not follow a pattern and the extent of skin involvement might range erratically from none to generalized body involvement. However, according to population surveys, most patients experience mild to moderate symptoms [70] and the percentage of patients reporting systemic therapies and/or hospitalization is no more than 20% [18].

The disease course is a bit unpredictable with spontaneous remissions and exacerbations with disease severity increasing in the winter and improving in the summer months. Again, there may be a disease flare up during sun exposure. The prevalence of photosensitive psoriasis according to a cross sectional survey was about 5.5% in patients who have type 1 skin, have a positive family history, in advanced age group and having psoriasis on their hands [71]. Moreover, psoriasis is reported to improve with pregnancy and aggravate during post partum period [72].

8. Differential diagnosis

The papulosquamous diseases which are considered in the differential diagnosis of psoriasis includes tinea infections, pityriasis rosea, and lichen planus. Psoriatic lesions are distinct from these entities being very well circumscribed, circular, red papules or plaques with a grey or silvery-white dry scale. In addition, psoriatic lesions are typically distributed symmetrically on the scalp, elbows, knees, lumbosacral area, and in the body folds. Psoriasis may develop at the site of trauma, known as Koebner's phenomenon.

Acute generalized exanthematic pustulosis, a self limiting febrile drug reaction usually resolving in 2 weeks after withdrawal of the suspected agent must be differentiated from generalized pustular psoriasis. Acute generalized exanthematic pustulosis is characterized by pinpoint nonfollicular pustules on erythematous patches mainly involving body folds, with single necrotic cells in epidermis, eosinophils and vasculitic changes in the dermis [73, 74].

9. To conclude

Psoriasis is an enigmatic disease involving a complex interplay of genetic, immunological and environmental factors. Advancement of science and technology has led to the identifications of many checkpoints in the disease course and pathology, which quite effectively has led to the development of novel therapeutic targets to limit disease progression. However, despite extensive research ino this disease the exact pathogenesis and clinical course of the disease is still unknown. Thus there is always a need for better diagnostic criteria, severity assessments and disease related Qol measures for determining long term outcomes of this elusive disease.

Acknowledgements

The images of clinical presentation of psoriasis are kind gifts from our mentor and eminent professor of Rheumatology and Dermatology, Dr. Siba P Raychaudhuri of University of California, Davis, CA, USA.

Author details

Ananya Datta Mitra[1,2] and Anupam Mitra[3*]

*Address all correspondence to: amitra@ucdavis.edu

1 Division of Rheumatology, Allergy and Clinical Immunology, University of California, Davis, School of Medicine, Sacramento, CA, USA

2 VA Medical Center Sacramento, Mather, CA, USA

3 Department of Dermatology, University of California, Davis, CA, USA. VA Medical Center Sacramento, Mather, CA, USA

References

[1] Raychaudhuri, S. P. A Cutting Edge Overview: Psoriatic Disease. *Clin Rev Allergy Immunol* 201

[2] Griffiths, C. E. Barker JN: Pathogenesis and clinical features of psoriasis. *Lancet* (2007).

[3] Mcdonald, C. J. Calabresi P: Psoriasis and occlusive vascular disease. *Br J Dermatol* (1978).

[4] Naldi, L, Chatenoud, L, & Linder, D. Belloni Fortina A, Peserico A, Virgili AR, Bruni PL, Ingordo V, Lo Scocco G, Solaroli C *et al*: Cigarette smoking, body mass index, and stressful life events as risk factors for psoriasis: results from an Italian case-control study. *J Invest Dermatol* (2005).

[5] Helliwell, P. S. Taylor WJ: Classification and diagnostic criteria for psoriatic arthritis. *Ann Rheum Dis* (2005). Suppl 2:ii, 3-8.

[6] Jobling, R. Naldi L: Assessing the impact of psoriasis and the relevance of qualitative research. *J Invest Dermatol* (2006).

[7] Li, K, & Armstrong, A. W. A review of health outcomes in patients with psoriasis. *Dermatol Clin* (2012). viii.

[8] Gudjonsson, J. E. Elder JT: Psoriasis: epidemiology. *Clin Dermatol* (2007).

[9] Bell, L. M, Sedlack, R, Beard, C. M, Perry, H. O, & Michet, C. J. Kurland LT: Incidence of psoriasis in Rochester, Minn, *Arch Dermatol* (1991)., 1980-1983.

[10] 10.Henseler, T. Christophers E: Psoriasis of early and late onset: characterization of two types of psoriasis vulgaris. *J Am Acad Dermatol* (1985).

[11] Raychaudhuri, S. P. Farber EM: The prevalence of psoriasis in the world. *J Eur Acad Dermatol Venereol* (2001).

[12] Farber EM NL: Epidemiology: natural history and genetics. *In:Roenigk Jr HH, Maibach HI, editorsNew York: Dekker 19981998*, 107-157.

[13] Chandran, V. Raychaudhuri SP: Geoepidemiology and environmental factors of psoriasis and psoriatic arthritis. *J Autoimmun* (2010). J, 314-321.

[14] Lin XR: Psoriasis in China. (1993). *J Dermatol.*

[15] Gelfand, J. M, Stern, R. S, Nijsten, T, Feldman, S. R, Thomas, J, Kist, J, & Rolstad, T. Margolis DJ: The prevalence of psoriasis in African Americans: results from a population-based study. *J Am Acad Dermatol* (2005).

[16] Naldi, L. Gambini D: The clinical spectrum of psoriasis. *Clin Dermatol* (2007).

[17] Naldi L: Epidemiology of psoriasis. (2004). *Curr Drug Targets Inflamm Allergy.*

[18] Naldi, L, Colombo, P, Placchesi, E. B, Piccitto, R, & Chatenoud, L. La Vecchia C: Study design and preliminary results from the pilot phase of the PraKtis study: self-reported diagnoses of selected skin diseases in a representative sample of the Italian population. *Dermatology* (2004).

[19] Langley, R. G, & Krueger, G. G. Griffiths CE: Psoriasis: epidemiology, clinical features, and quality of life. *Ann Rheum Dis* (2005). Suppl 2:iidiscussion ii24-15., 18-23.

[20] Naldi, L, Peli, L, & Parazzini, F. Carrel CF: Family history of psoriasis, stressful life events, and recent infectious disease are risk factors for a first episode of acute guttate psoriasis: results of a case-control study. *J Am Acad Dermatol* (2001).

[21] Martin, B. A, & Chalmers, R. J. Telfer NR: How great is the risk of further psoriasis following a single episode of acute guttate psoriasis? *Arch Dermatol* (1996).

[22] Sagoo, G. S, Tazi-ahnini, R, Barker, J. W, Elder, J. T, Nair, R. P, Samuelsson, L, Traupe, H, Trembath, R. C, & Robinson, D. A. Iles MM: Meta-analysis of genome-wide studies of psoriasis susceptibility reveals linkage to chromosomes 6and 4q28-q31 in Caucasian and Chinese Hans population. *J Invest Dermatol* (2004). , 21.

[23] Asumalahti, K, Ameen, M, Suomela, S, Hagforsen, E, Michaelsson, G, Evans, J, Munro, M, Veal, C, Allen, M, & Leman, J. Genetic analysis of PSORS1 distinguishes guttate psoriasis and palmoplantar pustulosis. *J Invest Dermatol* (2003).

[24] Kawada, A, Tezuka, T, Nakamizo, Y, Kimura, H, Nakagawa, H, Ohkido, M, Ozawa, A, Ohkawara, A, Kobayashi, H, & Harada, S. A survey of psoriasis patients in Japan from (1982). to 2001. *J Dermatol Sci* 2003, 31(1):59-64.

[25] Ohkawara, A, Yasuda, H, Kobayashi, H, Inaba, Y, Ogawa, H, & Hashimoto, I. Imamura S: Generalized pustular psoriasis in Japan: two distinct groups formed by differences in symptoms and genetic background. *Acta Derm Venereol* (1996).

[26] Zelickson, B. D. Muller SA: Generalized pustular psoriasis. A review of 63 cases. *Arch Dermatol* (1991).

[27] Viguier, M, Allez, M, Zagdanski, A. M, Bertheau, P, De Kerviler, E, Rybojad, M, Morel, P, Dubertret, L, & Lemann, M. Bachelez H: High frequency of cholestasis in generalized pustular psoriasis: Evidence for neutrophilic involvement of the biliary tract. *Hepatology* (2004).

[28] Oumeish, O. Y. Parish JL: Impetigo herpetiformis. *Clin Dermatol* (2006).

[29] Rosenberg, B. E. Strober BE: Acrodermatitis continua. *Dermatol Online J* (2004).

[30] Doherty, O. CJ, MacIntyre C: Palmoplantar pustulosis and smoking. *Br Med J (Clin Res Ed)* (1985).

[31] Kasperczyk, A. Freyschmidt J: Pustulotic arthroosteitis: spectrum of bone lesions with palmoplantar pustulosis. *Radiology* (1994).

[32] Szanto, E. Linse U: Arthropathy associated with palmoplantar pustulosis. *Clin Rheumatol* (1991).

[33] Hayem, G, Bouchaud-chabot, A, Benali, K, Roux, S, Palazzo, E, Silbermann-hoffman, O, & Kahn, M. F. Meyer O: SAPHO syndrome: a long-term follow-up study of 120 cases. *Semin Arthritis Rheum* (1999).

[34] Balasubramaniam, P. Berth-Jones J: Erythroderma: 90% skin failure. *Hosp Med* (2004).

[35] Salomon, J, & Szepietowski, J. C. Proniewicz A: Psoriatic nails: a prospective clinical study. *J Cutan Med Surg* (2003).

[36] Augustin, M, Reich, K, Glaeske, G, & Schaefer, I. Radtke M: Co-morbidity and age-related prevalence of psoriasis: Analysis of health insurance data in Germany. *Acta Derm Venereol* (2010).

[37] Tsai, T. F, Wang, T. S, Hung, S. T, Tsai, P. I, Schenkel, B, & Zhang, M. Tang CH: Epidemiology and comorbidities of psoriasis patients in a national database in Taiwan. *J Dermatol Sci* (2011).

[38] Alamanos, Y, & Voulgari, P. V. Drosos AA: Incidence and prevalence of psoriatic arthritis: a systematic review. *J Rheumatol* (2008).

[39] Gladman, D. D, Shuckett, R, Russell, M. L, & Thorne, J. C. Schachter RK: Psoriatic arthritis (PSA)--an analysis of 220 patients. *Q J Med* (1987).

[40] Jones, S. M, Armas, J. B, Cohen, M. G, Lovell, C. R, & Evison, G. McHugh NJ: Psoriatic arthritis: outcome of disease subsets and relationship of joint disease to nail and skin disease. *Br J Rheumatol* (1994).

[41] Torre Alonso JCRodriguez Perez A, Arribas Castrillo JM, Ballina Garcia J, Riestra Noriega JL, Lopez Larrea C: Psoriatic arthritis (PA): a clinical, immunological and radiological study of 180 patients. *Br J Rheumatol* (1991).

[42] Madland, T. M, Apalset, E. M, Johannessen, A. E, & Rossebo, B. Brun JG: Prevalence, disease manifestations, and treatment of psoriatic arthritis in Western Norway. *J Rheumatol* (2005).

[43] Zisman, D, Eder, L, Elias, M, Laor, A, Bitterman, H, Rozenbaum, M, Feld, J, & Rimar, D. Rosner I: Clinical and demographic characteristics of patients with psoriatic arthritis in northern Israel. *Rheumatol Int* (2012).

[44] Michet, C. J, & Mason, T. G. Mazlumzadeh M: Hip joint disease in psoriatic arthritis: risk factors and natural history. *Ann Rheum Dis* (2005).

[45] Taylor, W, Gladman, D, Helliwell, P, Marchesoni, A, & Mease, P. Mielants H: Classification criteria for psoriatic arthritis: development of new criteria from a large international study. *Arthritis Rheum* (2006).

[46] Nossent, J. C. Gran JT: Epidemiological and clinical characteristics of psoriatic arthritis in northern Norway. *Scand J Rheumatol* (2009).

[47] Moll, J. M. Wright V: Psoriatic arthritis. *Semin Arthritis Rheum* (1973).

[48] Naldi, L. Chatenoud L: [Psoriasis and cancer: more than a chance link]. *Ann Dermatol Venereol* (2006).

[49] Henseler, T. Christophers E: Disease concomitance in psoriasis. *J Am Acad Dermatol* (1995).

[50] Neimann, A. L, Shin, D. B, Wang, X, Margolis, D. J, & Troxel, A. B. Gelfand JM: Prevalence of cardiovascular risk factors in patients with psoriasis. *J Am Acad Dermatol* (2006).

[51] Esposito, M, Saraceno, R, Giunta, A, & Maccarone, M. Chimenti S: An Italian study on psoriasis and depression. *Dermatology* (2006).

[52] Sommer, D. M, Jenisch, S, Suchan, M, & Christophers, E. Weichenthal M: Increased prevalence of the metabolic syndrome in patients with moderate to severe psoriasis. *Arch Dermatol Res* (2006).

[53] Gelfand, J. M, Neimann, A. L, Shin, D. B, Wang, X, & Margolis, D. J. Troxel AB: Risk of myocardial infarction in patients with psoriasis. *JAMA* (2006).

[54] Mallbris, L, Akre, O, Granath, F, Yin, L, Lindelof, B, & Ekbom, A. Stahle-Backdahl M: Increased risk for cardiovascular mortality in psoriasis inpatients but not in outpatients. *Eur J Epidemiol* (2004).

[55] Kimball, A. B, Jacobson, C, Weiss, S, & Vreeland, M. G. Wu Y: The psychosocial burden of psoriasis. *Am J Clin Dermatol* (2005).

[56] Gelfand, J. M, Troxel, A. B, Lewis, J. D, Kurd, S. K, Shin, D. B, Wang, X, & Margolis, D. J. Strom BL: The risk of mortality in patients with psoriasis: results from a population-based study. *Arch Dermatol* (2007).

[57] Mcgowan, J. W, Pearce, D. J, Chen, J, Richmond, D, & Balkrishnan, R. Feldman SR: The skinny on psoriasis and obesity. *Arch Dermatol* (2005).

[58] Lindegard B: Diseases associated with psoriasis in a general population of 159middle-aged, urban, native Swedes. *Dermatologica* (1986).

[59] Prodanovich, S, Ma, F, Taylor, J. R, Pezon, C, & Fasihi, T. Kirsner RS: Methotrexate reduces incidence of vascular diseases in veterans with psoriasis or rheumatoid arthritis. *J Am Acad Dermatol* (2005).

[60] Choi, H. K, Hernan, M. A, Seeger, J. D, & Robins, J. M. Wolfe F: Methotrexate and mortality in patients with rheumatoid arthritis: a prospective study. *Lancet* (2002).

[61] Farber, E. M. Nall ML: The natural history of psoriasis in 5,600 patients. *Dermatologica* (1974).

[62] Schmitt, J. Wozel G: The psoriasis area and severity index is the adequate criterion to define severity in chronic plaque-type psoriasis. *Dermatology* (2005).

[63] Wilson, I. B. Cleary PD: Linking clinical variables with health-related quality of life. A conceptual model of patient outcomes. *JAMA* (1995).

[64] Katz S: The science of quality of life. (1987). *J Chronic Dis.*

[65] Finlay AY: Quality of life measurement in dermatology: a practical guide. (1997). *Br J Dermatol.*

[66] Neill, O, & Kelly, P. P: Postal questionnaire study of disability in the community associated with psoriasis. *BMJ* (1996).

[67] guidance ECfPMPNftreatment ociompift, (2454). opCE.

[68] Adams, K. F, Schatzkin, A, Harris, T. B, Kipnis, V, Mouw, T, Ballard-barbash, R, & Hollenbeck, A. Leitzmann MF: Overweight, obesity, and mortality in a large prospective cohort of persons 50 to 71 years old. *N Engl J Med* (2006).

[69] Unaeze, J, Nijsten, T, Murphy, A, & Ravichandran, C. Stern RS: Impact of psoriasis on health-related quality of life decreases over time: an year prospective study. *J Invest Dermatol* (2006). , 11.

[70] Gelfand, J. M, Feldman, S. R, Stern, R. S, Thomas, J, & Rolstad, T. Margolis DJ: Determinants of quality of life in patients with psoriasis: a study from the US population. *J Am Acad Dermatol* (2004).

[71] Ros, A. M. Eklund G: Photosensitive psoriasis. An epidemiologic study. *J Am Acad Dermatol* (1987). Pt 1):752-758.

[72] Dunna, S. F. Finlay AY: Psoriasis: improvement during and worsening after pregnancy. *Br J Dermatol* (1989).

[73] Saissi, E. H, Beau-salinas, F, Jonville-bera, A. P, & Lorette, G. Autret-Leca E: [Drugs associated with acute generalized exanthematic pustulosis]. *Ann Dermatol Venereol* (2003).

[74] Sidoroff, A, Halevy, S, Bavinck, J. N, & Vaillant, L. Roujeau JC: Acute generalized exanthematous pustulosis (AGEP)--a clinical reaction pattern. *J Cutan Pathol* (2001).

Section 2

Causes of Psoriasis

Chapter 3

Psoriasis as a Chess Board — An Update of Psoriasis Pathophysiology

Robyn S Fallen, Anupam Mitra, Laura Morrisey and Hermenio Lima

Additional information is available at the end of the chapter

http://dx.doi.org/10.5772/53580

1. Introduction

By virtue of the dynamic nature of the scientific process, the description of the pathogenesis of a disease is always a work in progress. Each day new research shapes and refines our understanding of disease processes; an attempt to describe the current scientific understanding provides merely a snapshot of a body of knowledge that is constantly changing. However, characterizing a disease using homeostatic and physiological terms allows the creation of a framework to convey the most up-to-date theories while maintaining the potential for their evolution.

The complex nature of psoriasis can similarly be unveiled through understanding the historical context of our current understanding, examining prevailing hypotheses, and extrapolating horizons for new research. To develop a framework for understanding the pathogenesis of psoriasis and its evolution, the first perception to be changed is the prevalent view of the immune system. The general notion of the immune system as a defense arrangement that protects us against the microorganisms must be changed. This view results from a reduction of the process itself and, as mentioned by Dr. Nelson Vaz, are features derived from the birth of the immunology [1]. Immunology, as a scientific field, is new in the history of medicine. Immunology developed in a century marked by the First and Second World War and Cold War tension. Hence, many models to exemplify the immunological concepts were simplified and described in relation to war affairs to facilitate the understanding of this science. In this model, if a microorganism attacks a human being, the individual advocates the use of the immune system to counteract. Another simple aspect is the teleology that prevails in the immune science. For example, the T lymphocyte exists to kill cells infected with intracellular parasites. This model full of logic and consequences does not apply in many other areas of medical and non-medical sciences. As such, it is necessary to move to a new approach to describing the relationship between the immune system and environment. In this new paradigm, the immune system does not react, but rather interacts with the environment, and this contact is made through the skin and mucous membranes. This interaction, causal or not, can have different results. In most cases, there is a balance, imperceptible to other sensory systems, which is characterized by the integrity of what we call health. Thus, homeostasis disorders or imbalances lead to disease. This seems obvious when written, but this search for stability has continuity for the duration of the life of a given organism. If we consider the immune system a sensorial system, it interacts with the modifications of the environment, detects this information of change, and responds with adjustments to maintain homeostasis. You might reduce this view by comparing it to an engine that runs under different types of fuel mixture. It detects the different fuel composition and changes the compression ratio of the cylinder for better efficiency to keep the car moving.

For better observation of this psoriasis pathogenesis, we will make a technical simulation of the immune system in a specific situation. This simulation will cover various aspects of immune response, spanning from the beginning of the inflammatory response, to specific immune response through the development of psoriasis. Here, under a historical perspective and comparing with a chess game, the main objective is to provide insights on the central role of some of these cytokines and immunological pathways in psoriasis pathophysiology. Through this, the aim is to explain some facts of modern immunodermatology that might be useful for clinicians to understand the basis of the immunology of psoriasis. Moreover, an important goal is to dispel some misinformation that might have a negative impact on the use of new immunomodulators and medications available for use by physicians. Treatment basis and therapeutic response experience strongly supports the use of immunomodulators as important modalities in the treatment of psoriatic arthritis and plaque psoriasis. Studies with these therapeutic agents, which act in different steps of the psoriatic inflammatory cascade, have also shown significant efficacy. [2].

Directly targeting this inflammatory cascade, blocking specific cytokines is a modern treatment option for psoriasis and other autoimmune diseases [3]. The rationale for this therapy arises from pathophysiology; in different autoimmune diseases there is an increase in production of proinflammatory cytokines by the immune system. Inflammatory cytokines, like many other cytokines, have an important role in both maintaining health and participating in disease manifestation [4]. This chapter discusses the pivotal role of some of these cytokines in psoriasis pathophysiology, how our understanding of its mechanism evolved, and how blocking the effect of a specific cytokine might substantially improve the disease condition.

2. Pre–biologic immunological history of psoriasis

Psoriasis is a common skin disease with extra-cutaneous manifestations. It is characterized by chronic inflammation of the skin with changes in the maturation of keratinocytes, which is manifested by the hyperproliferation of the epidermis. Moreover, inflammatory reaction can be found in other systems of the same patient. However, this disease is mediated by T lymphocytes, orchestrated by orchestration multigenic and environmental factors. The altered immune system is essential for the inflammation present in both the skin and other organs. A concept of a multi-systemic disorder involving different organs of the patient and reflects a better understanding of the complex pathophysiology of this disease [2].

The concept of biological therapy for psoriasis has been derived from its etiopathogenesis. As in a chess game, these new forms of treatment have evolved from an integration of the knowledge of interactions between the immune system cells (pieces) and its cytokines (movements) that initiates the pathologic processes and ultimately leads to the development of the clinical features of psoriasis.

In ancient records, the initial causes of psoriasis were attributed to multiple sources ranging from the divine power to racial associations [5]. An unknown infectious organism was indicated as a source of psoriasis in 1927 [6]. Later, its etiology was described as primarily and essentially an epidermal problem, independent of immunologic phenomena [7]. The main objective of cytotoxic drugs developed in the 20th century, such as methotrexate, was to reduce keratinocyte proliferation. Immunological studies on psoriatic patients identified changes in humoral immune reactions as part of the overall problem but not the cause [8, 9]. Efficacy of the cytotoxic drugs in the late 1960s paved the road for ideas about the role of the immune system in psoriasis [10, 11]. Further investigations in the 1970s revealed the role of immunologic factors in psoriasis. However, the dominant thought was that psoriasis was a disease of faulty epidermopoiesis due to impaired autocontrol mechanisms [12]. Hunter et al. wrote "More work on cell turnover and its regulation will give the clue to psoriasis" [13].

Other studies in the 1970s revealed the role of immunologic factors in psoriasis. Histopathologic examination of psoriatic lesions showed a striking resemblance to cellular inflammatory reactions observed in allergic contact dermatitis [14]. A selective immunosuppressant effect was the initial hypothesis used to describe the pathological cellular immune response [15]. Soon thereafter, the discovery of a soluble factor that played an important role in keratinocyte proliferation helped to form the cytokine-based theory for the induction/maintenance of the inflammatory and proliferative cascades of psoriatic lesions [16]. Subsequently, an integrated theory explaining the etiopathogenesis of psoriasis came into play: in a genetically susceptible patient, immunological factors trigger rapid turnover in the epidermis resulting in the development of psoriasis [17].

The fundamental confirmation that any defect of the skin is not sufficient by itself to maintain a psoriatic lesion occurred in the subsequent decade. Some studies confirmed that T cells and soluble factors could stimulate keratinocyte proliferation. Immunophenotyping of psoriatic lesions showed mixed T lymphocyte (TL) cell populations (CD4 and CD8) and Langerhans cells (LCs) distinct from normal skin [18]. This cellular infiltrate changed with topical or systemic treatment [19, 20]. In another study, failure of plasma exchange and leukapheresis ruled out the major participation of humoral immune system in the pathogenesis of psoriasis [21]. Thus, the cellular arm of the immune system was implicated in psoriasis for the first time during the 1980s [22].

During the 1990s, research on immunopathogenesis of psoriasis thus focused on the cellular and the cytokine components of the immune system. Researchers observed that an influx of activated T lymphocytes, mainly CD4+, HLA-DR+, Interleukin (IL)-2 receptor - CD25+ T cells, was one of the earliest events of psoriasis [23]. Based on Mosmman and Coffman's publication [24], these T lymphocytes were classified as T helper (Th) type 1 cytokine producers (Th1) [25]. They produce Interferon (IFN)-γ, IL-2, and Tumor Necrosis Factor (TNF)-α cytokines and implied that a cellular type 1 reaction was responsible for psoriasis (Figure 1). The observation of the historical evolution of the extra-cutaneous manifestations of psoriasis and their pathogenesis confirms the idea of a multi-organ disease with complex immunological pathways [2].

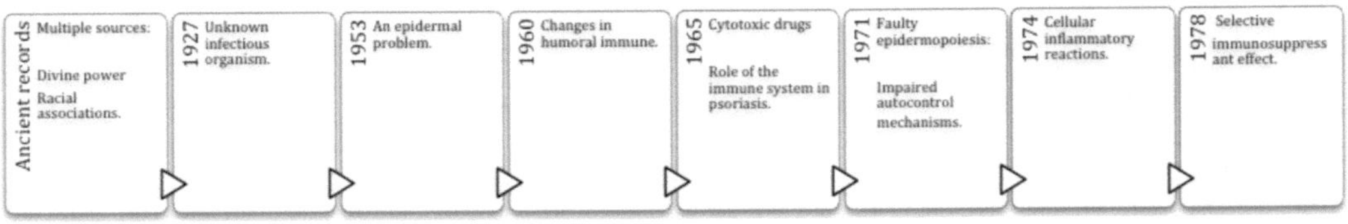

Figure 1. Time line of development of psoriasis pathophysiology: From unknown to epidermal problem through Immunological disease.

3. Psoriasis: Many pieces and movements on a complex chessboard

Psoriasis plaque is induced and maintained by multiple interactions between cells of the skin and immune system. It seems that the pathogenesis of psoriasis could involve a stage of cellular infiltration resulting in epidermal (keratinocyte) proliferation. Each inflammatory pathway (IL-12/Th1, IL-23/Th17, and IL-22/Th22) has its impact on psoriasis development [26]. The different pathways are based on the fact that T helper cells can be skewed towards mutually exclusive subtypes on the basis of the cytokine environment [27, 28]. The process of T lymphocyte reactivation results from interaction of T cells with the resident antigen presenting cells (APCs) found in plaque psoriasis, which in turn determines the cytokine environment and Th1/Th17/Th22 pathway.

The primary etiopathogenesis of an autoimmune disease, or the activation of Th1/Th17/Th22 pathways, is the dysregulation of immune system activation since the development of autoreactive lymphocytes occurs in the same basic manner as lymphocyte activation. The understanding of this process or processes is very important to maintain the balance of the normal performance of the immune system. Briefly, it is comparable to the process to find the moment where one player lost the chess game based on the retroactive analysis of his moves. Cytokines are the possible moves of different pieces of the game. Many pieces can produce the same movement but with different results. The moves are the key players in generating or establishing a specific immune system reaction. Therefore, blocking cytokines that maintain autoimmune activity has become one the most successful strategies for autoimmunity therapy. A new balance can be established with the removal of a key piece or blocking of a lethal move so that the critical players are removed from the chessboard of an autoimmune response.

As with any other disease involving the immune system, psoriatic manifestation begins with Antigen-Presenting Cells (APC) activation by an unknown trigger. Different factors including infections, trauma, medications, and emotional stress can initiate the initial phase of the disease. Such factors can activate keratinocytes to release cytokines such as IL-1 and TNF-α, initiating the effector phase of psoriasis by activating resident skin macrophages and Dendritic Cells (DCs). DCs migrate to the regional lymph node, which initiates T lymphocyte activation in response to the stimuli. This is part of the working model of the immune synapse of T cells in psoriasis, integrating T cell signaling pathways in autoimmunity [29]. This association leads to the production of IL-12/Th1/IFN-γ pathway. Many molecules in the plasma membrane of both cells, other than the Major Histocompatibility Complex (MHC) and T Cell Receptor (TCR), are involved in this phase and can be used as a target molecule for the treatment of psoriasis. The most important molecules are ICAM-1, LFA-3, and CD80/CD86 in the DC and LFA-1, CD2, and CD28 in the T cell, respectively. Alefacept, a fusion protein used for psoriasis treatment, blocks T cells activation by interfering with CD2 on the T cell membrane, thereby blocking the costimulatory molecule LFA-3/CD2 interaction [30]. Furthermore, it has recently been discovered that IL-27 suppressed macrophage responses to TNF-α and IL-1β, thus identifying an anti-inflammatory function of IL-27 [31].

Continuing the evolving complex immunological chess game, the activated T lymphocyte Th1 cytokine producers leave the lymph node and migrate to the skin where cytokines like TNF-α, produced by keratinocytes and activated DCs, facilitate T lymphocyte diapedesis into the dermis and epidermis [32]. The TNF-α induces the skin immune cell infiltration by inducing chemokines and upregulating adhesion molecules on the endothelial cells of dermal vessels. Adhesion molecules such as CLA and LFA-1 on the T lymphocyte membrane and E-selectin and ICAM-1 on the endothelial cell membrane are involved in this process. Efalizumab, a Humanized Anti-CD11a, Anti-LFA-1 molecule has been used in psoriasis treatment by blocking the TL migration to the skin [33]. In summary, dendritic cells and effector T-cells are important in the development of the psoriatic lesion, and cytokines produced by these cells stimulate keratinocytes to proliferate and increase the migration of inflammatory cells into the skin, promoting epidermal hyperplasia and inflammation [34].

3.1. Chessboard: The skin's influence on psoriasis development

The primary cause of psoriasis has not been not found. Factors such as genetics and environmental exposure are now recognized to play a role in psoriasis development. Certainly, autoimmunity does not appear to be the only, or necessary, component to the development of psoriasis. However, psoriasis is a manifestation of skin immune reactions. Inflammation is a key feature of pathogenesis, with all inflammatory cell types implicated in psoriasis pathology by multiple interactions between cells of the skin or from other organs and the immune system. Nonetheless, the etiology of psoriasis as an epidermal problem or a disease of faulty epidermopoiesis due to impaired autocontrol mechanisms is not completely wrong. Keratinocyte-derived inflammatory molecules ampliy skin immune responses associated with psoriasis, and contribute to the disease process and clinical phenotype [35]. Psoriatic keratinocytes respond aberrantly to cytokines and show altered intracellular signaling pathways [36].

Heterogeneous functions of other skin resident cells, such as fibroblasts and endothelial cells, may also contribute to the pathogenesis of psoriasis [37]. Furthermore, leukocytes that infiltrate skin lesions have been shown to be involved in the pathogenesis of this disease [38]. Despite parallels to the chicken and egg causality dilemma, all of these contribute to the presentation in patients suffering from psoriasis that is later observed by clinicians.

3.2. Immunopathogenesis of psoriasis is a teleological model

From the previous data, it is well known that the immunopathogenesis of psoriasis is complex. It involves alterations in the innate and acquired immunologic system. In the most accepted models, cells of the skin when activated produce immunological mediators that act upon the cells of the specific immune system. The action is amplified by the opposite direction [39].

The most studied theories about autoimmune disease etiology associate the immune dysregulation and loss of tolerance due to the impact of environmental factors on genetically susceptible individuals. The literature has always highlighted the importance of the microorganism in the lack of immune homeostasis in psoriasis. The linkage of antigens of infectious agents to the toll like receptors can activate keratinocytes and other cells to release innumerous chemokines, cytokines and growth factors. Activated keratinocytes are capable of recruiting and activating T cells. Therefore, infections are considered an important component that can unleash the manifestation of psoriasis[40].

3.3. Dissociation between immunopathogenesis and immunological concepts

In accordance to the actual immunopathogenesis models for psoriasis, the skin is the body's primary defense against external invasion. However, the keratinocytes, in defending the body against the microorganism, induces the migration of cutaneous lymphocyte-associated antigen (CLA) positive T cells. Finally, T cells play a central role in initiating and perpetuating the immunological mechanisms of psoriasis [41].

In this context, the possibility arises that endogenous, normal, housekeeping self-proteins might be epitopic targets in autoimmune responses in psoriasis. The transition from self-reactivity to the autoimmune pathology appears to be mediated by a complex network of overlapping phenomena [42]. However, all studies about the antigen identification in psoriasis, like in many other autoimmune diseases, did not find an optimal autoantigen for studying the relationship between similarity level and immune responses [43].

Therefore, the actual models of immunopathogenesis of psoriasis break the specificity basic statement of immunology. There are historical reasons for the dissociation between immunopathogenesis models and immunology concepts. Immunology emerged as a biomedical science, concerned with host defense and production of anti-infectious vaccines. Ehrlich's side-chain theory explained the anti-infectious protection granted by vaccines and serotherapy [44]. It was the first steps of the development of initial cognitive metaphors, such as recognition and memory.

The clonal selective theory of antibody formation in the 1950s was a new evolution and the initiation of neo-Darwinism in Immunology. The selective theories of antibody formation resulted from the union of Immunology with Darwin's theory of evolution. They also amplified the "Defensive metaphors". Lymphocytes are supposed to respond specifically to stimuli. Except for brief moments of activating or inhibiting interactions, lymphocytes are believed to act independently from each other. Therefore, the immune system defends the body by amplification of specific lymphocytes.

3.4. Defensive metaphor

In seeking to understand the unknown, mysterious, or abstract, the human mind draws comparisons to the known, familiar, and concrete. When these comparisons are made explicit, we call them metaphors or analogies. Scientists draw on metaphors when struggling with phenomena that defy easy observation, such as the immune system. Immunology developed many metaphors based on the scenario of its development. The naissance of immunology was marked by the great World Wars and the Cold War tension. Consequently, immunological concepts were simplified and described as war affairs.

The war metaphor for the immune response is appealing, in part, because it seems to create a deeper understanding of the rules that direct the immune system actions. The consequence of immunologists' fondness for war metaphors, the authentication of the models has hardly been tapped. However, any metaphors used to explain the immune system evoke intuitive notions of strategy, skill and competition. Rarely do they indicate a deep understanding of the particular clinical variation present in the arenas of medical life.

The underlying principle in this framework is the immune system as a "defense system." When it is said that the immune system defends the body, there is the use, intentionally or not, of a metaphor. This is also a teleological argument (from the Greek τέλος for "end", "purpose", or "goal"). Teleological argument is a knowledge or explanation about a fact that relates to a final question. Teleological reasoning is an anthropomorphic interpretation used in science. Therefore, it is given that there is an end or a function for the biological being or immune system. However, there is not much teleological argument in physics or other natural science fields. Do you know any reason why the earth gravitates around the sun?

Immunologists are in a comparable position to use metaphors inasmuch as the cellular and molecular relationships that form the immune response are things that cannot readily be seen. Famous and basilar modern immunological metaphors include viewing the immune system as a planning body at a multidimensional space in which the lymphocytes are developing defensive strategies against invaders or irritants. Another side of this favorite metaphor is that of the main reason why bacteria invade the bodies is because those bodies harbor environments where the bacteria can survive and multiply. The immune system protects the body from invaders like bacteria, viruses and parasites.

There are consequences to this metaphor interpretation. The immune system does not act as one structure or system. A system is described as a collection of elements connected to each other in such a way that acting upon one element has repercussions upon all the others. Lymphocytes are supposed to respond independently specifically to antigen stimuli. Therefore, lymphocytes do not interact with the organism or with other lymphocytes. They are clonal units. Thus, lymphocytes cannot organize themselves in a system.

In the actual stage of the clonal selection theory acceptance and consequent metaphor interpretation, the proposition of significantly different concepts or description of the immune system have been excluded from the scientific media. The net result of such a theoretic narrowness is the characterization of a massive variety of cellular or molecular independent components involved in immunological activity. Therefore, the expansion, contraction and regulation of specific clones of lymphocytes are insufficient to generate all known immunological phenomena. Finally, the lack of a different view about the immune system followed in a flagrant inability to create new vaccines, to understand and treat allergies or autoimmune diseases as psoriasis.

3.5. Game theory as a new proposal for immunopathogenesis of psoriasis

Does the interpretation of the data in immunology, as it is today, represent the only possible way to have an immune response? Is there a new model where the immune system can be explained and the immunopathogenesis of autoimmune diseases as psoriasis can be interpreted? This is a logical question that should follow the previous assumptions.

Consistent with the position that the details of a immune response matter, any other proposition begins by reviewing and incorporating the accepted rules, constraints, and properties available for the immune system - the Immunology game's inner logic. The application of game theory to Immunology thinking is our new proposition to explain autoimmune diseases and other immunologic responses. The objective here is to begin taking games seriously as potential sources of insight into the relationship that determines the Immune system.

Game theory is a set of concepts aimed at decision making in situations of competition and conflict, as well as of cooperation and interdependence, under specified rules [45]. Game theory metaphors began with the idea regarding the existence of mixed-strategy towards equilibrium. The discordant note of this view of game theory with the actual immunological response is the prevailing opinion among game theorists that any interaction will eventually converge to Nash equilibrium predictions under the right conditions. Although the initial application of game theory to immunology does not involve any of the requirements of the Nash equilibrium, the human homeostasis conforms nicely to predictions of the Nash equilibrium or relevant refinement. Absence of homeostasis or disease is the lack of stability in the immune system concept.

Researchers are starting to realize that this simplistic view of the immune system as defensive system needs a radical rethink [46]. The focus has been less on equilibria that correspond to a notion of rationality or teleologism, but rather on ones that would be maintained by evolutionary forces. In this new view, the skin has no longer been thought of as a mere physical barrier to attack by pathogens. Recent studies suggest the interplay between the skin's resident microorganisms, known collectively as the skin microbiome, and immune mediated organ-specific diseases [47]. Increasingly, it has been recognized that disruptions in the commensal microflora may lead to immune dysfunction and autoimmunity. Therefore, the microbiome influence the host's immune system [48]. In particular, there are new findings on the role of the microbiome in psoriasis [49].

Biologists have used game theory. The known game theory equilibrium in biology is the evolutionarily stable strategy (ESS) [50]. Additionally, biologists have used evolutionary game theory and the ESS to explain many seemingly incongruous phenomena in nature. Paradoxically, it has turned out that game theory is more applied to biology than to the field of immunology for which it can be an evolutionary metaphor. Considering some of the ways in which game metaphors have been used in biology analysis, observing that most game metaphors involve only vague and fleeting references to some generic game with the goal of making a preconceived point. We contrast this with analogies in the natural sciences, in which knowledge of a well-understood phenomenon is used to shed light on another that is less well understood. A new idea has to propose a nonteleological view including all possible natural evolutions, which will necessarily generate other set of problems and enigmas. A nonteleolcgical thinking is a way of viewing things as they are, rather than seeking explanations for them [51]. However, the practicality of a nonteleological view in immunology is null nowadays [45].

In summary, although the costs of infections to immune system are meaningful, a growing body of evidence supports a general benefit associated with infectivity. Reducing the risk of uncontrolled inflammation and limiting the tissue damage caused by injury are important features of host defense against pathogens, but would be beneficial in a variety of autoimmune diseases [52]. Game theory may help to appreciate the benefits of immunity to infection. This is the challenge for the new homeostatic immune system metaphors that explain the autoimmunity mechanisms as in psoriasis.

4. The initial biologic treatments for psoriasis and implications for the understanding of immunological mechanism of psoriasis

Psoriasis was defined as Th1 type of disease based on the early understanding of the T helper subsets. The initial belief was that infiltrating T cell subpopulations derived from the draining lymph node regulated the development of the inflammatory responses in the skin by producing IFN-γ and TNF-α [53]. The Th1-derived cytokines produced by these infiltrating Th1 favors further Th1 cell access, upregulates keratinocyte chemokine production, and supports dermal DC myeloid type (DC11c+) activation. In response to this cytokine activation, keratinocytes and other cells produce a plethora of immune mediators, which induce and amplify inflammatory responses in the skin [54].

As a result, two logical biologic therapeutic approaches were tested: one was the administration of counter regulatory type 2 cytokines and the second was the blocking of type 1 cytokines. The use of monoclonal antibodies or fusion proteins to neutralize cytokines started to be used on a large scale because of their efficacy and practicality.

These studies have proved to be a useful biological model and test ground for evaluation of the skin immune system and psoriasis. Although these drugs were not initially developed in the treatment of psoriasis, but rather in rheumatoid arthritis and Crohn's disease, the observation that Crohn's disease patients with psoriasis were improving while on anti-TNF therapy profoundly influenced the studies that were to come [55].

Although clinical response to anti-TNF suggested a role for Th1 cells in psoriasis, evidence coming from other studies demonstrated that Th1/Th2 paradigm and key role of TNF were not sufficient to explain the full pathogenesis of psoriasis. At this point some academic resistance to an immunological pathogenesis for psoriasis was raised [56]. However, the main interpretation was that an important piece of the immunological cytokine puzzle was missing. Many other pieces would be involved in such a complex game.

5. The IL–12/23 and its role in the immunopathogenesis psoriasis

The initial quest for the missing cytokines was the search for pathway inducers. Researchers first noted that IL-12 is crucial for Th1-cell differentiation [57]. IL-12 signaling via its receptor activates Stat4 (signal transducer and activator of transcription 4), which upregulates IFN-γ. IFN-γ activates Stat1, which enhance T-bet (T-box expressed in T cells), the leading TH1 transcription factor, further enhancing IFN- γ production and downregulating IL-4 and IL-5 expression [58]. IFN-γ mediates many of the pro-inflammatory activities of IL-12. Phagocytes and Dendritic Cells (DCs) are the main producers of IL-12 in response to microbial stimulation [59], and this relationship links innate resistance and adaptive immunity. The main function of IL-12 is resistance to infections with bacteria and intracellular parasites. However, it plays an important role in the Th1 response that sustains organ-specific autoimmunity [60]. The use of anti-IL-12 mAb (monoclonal antibody) in an experimental model of psoriasis also suggested the therapeutic value of blocking IL-12 in humans [61], although side effects of the drug limited further development in this area.

For many years, the IL-12-dependent Th1 cells were thought to be essential for the induction of autoimmunity. However, during the Th1/Th2 paradigm studies, an IFN-γ-independent mechanism responsible for the pathogenesis of many inflammatory diseases and psoriasis was found [62]. IL-12 and IL-23, as discovered previously from human DNA sequence information, share the subunit p40 [63]. The use of anti-IL-12/23p40 and anti-IFN mAb ultimately established at least part of the solution to the riddle. Only neutralization of p40, but not of IFN-γ, ameliorated chronic inflammatory reactions. This finding suggested that the latter cytokine, IL-23, accounted for the IFN-γ-independent mechanism of inflammation.

Identified from human DNA sequence information, IL-23, like IL-12, is also a heterodimeric cytokine composed of the same subunit p40 paired with the unique p19 [64]. It has been reported that IL-12 and IL-23 are up-regulated in psoriatic skin [65]. Human studies with anti-IL-12p40 have shown that this treatment not only ameliorates psoriasis, but also down-regulates type 1 cytokines and IL-12/IL-23 in lesional skin [66]. Besides sharing the subunit p40 and signaling through similar receptors, IL-23 and IL-12 are responsible for driving different T-cell subsets. Moreover, presence of abundant IL-23^{+} dendritic cells as well as elevated mRNA expression for both subunits of IL-23 (IL-23p19 and IL-23p40) in psoriatic lesions supports the role of IL-23 in the pathogenesis of psoriasis [65, 67-69]. Genetic studies have revealed that polymorphisms in IL-23p19, IL-12/23p40, and IL-23R are associated with increased risk of psoriasis [70-72]. Furthermore, in an animal xenograft model of psoriasis, Tonel G et al showed that treatment with anti human IL-23 mAb causes statistically significant reduction of acanthosis and papillomatosis index in grafts of mice in comparison to isotype controlled mice. Moreover, they found comparable efficacy of anti human IL-23 mAb with anti TNF-α (infliximab) in blocking the development of psoriasis. They also showed a significant decrease in CD3+ T cells mainly in the epidermis of mice treated with anti human IL-23 mAb in comparison to control mice [73].

IL-23 could also mediate and sustain late-stage chronic inflammation by the production of IL-17 by Th17 [74]. IL-23 plays an important role as a central growth factor [75-77]. In presence of TGF-β and IL-6, IL-23 helps in development of Th17 cells whereas TGF-β is inhibitory to production of IL-22 [78-80] (Figure 2).

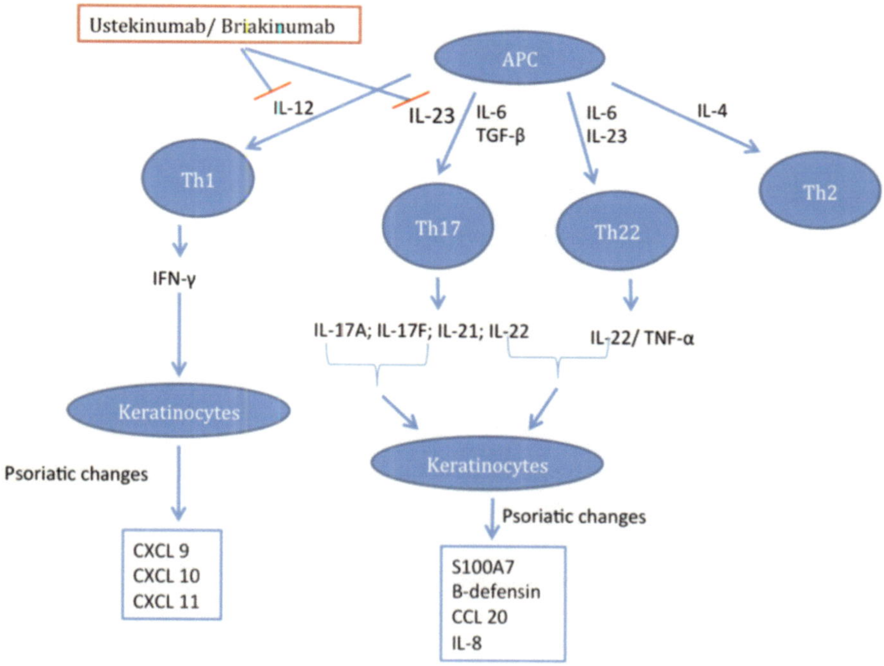

Figure 2. The pivotal role of some of IL-12 and IL-23 in psoriasis etiopathogenesis: How blocking the effects of these cytokines substantially improve the disease condition.

The IL-23/Th17/IL-17 immune axis was initially elucidated when IL-17 gene expression was induced by *B. burgdorferi* independent of IL-12 [81]. The IL-17–producing CD4+ T cells distinct from those producing either IL-4 or IFN-γ were called Th17 [82]. Patients with psoriasis have increased Th17 cells as well as increased expression of mRNA for Th17 cytokines (IL-17A; IL-17F; TNF-α; IL-21 and IL-22) and chemokines (CCL20) [83-87]. In psoriasis, Th17 cytokine IL-17A mainly induces cytokine and chemokine production by keratinocytes [84, 88, 89], whereas IL-22 induces proliferation of keratinocytes and production of antimicrobial peptides by keratinocytes [78, 90-92]. The role of IL-23 and IL-17 in psoriasis was further substantiated in some animal studies with recombinant IL-23 and anti IL-17A. In wild type (WT) mice, injection of recombinant murine (rm) IL-23 induces epidermal hyperplasia [93, 94], whereas, in IL-17 -/- mice showed less epidermal hyperplasia after repeated injection of rmIL-23. A recent publication by Rizzo et al showed that WT mice do not show epidermal hyperplasia to injection of rmIL-23 if they were treated with anti IL-17A antibodies [95]. A redundant cytokine model has emerged as the evolving explanation for psoriasis pathogenesis. It is based on the IL-12/Th1/ IFN-γ - TNF-α and the IL-23/Th17/IL-17 immune pathways (Figure 3). The effectiveness of the anti-TNF treatment of psoriasis validated the first axis. The efficacy of anti-p40 (anti-IL12/23) treatment confirms the other [96].

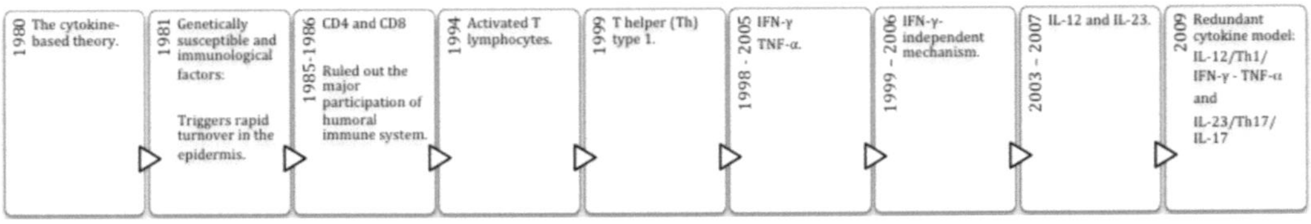

Figure 3. Time line of development of psoriasis pathophysiology: From complex immunological disease through genetic participation until recent advances.

6. Selective IL–23/Th17/IL–17 immune axis inhibition

IL-23 favors the proliferation of the Th17 subtype and consequent production of IL-22 and IL-6 that stimulates the proliferation of keratinocytes. IL-17 favors infiltration of neutrophils into the skin forming the typical Munro's micro-abscesses with some participation of IL-22 [97].

Studies have demonstrated that anti-p40 (anti-IL-12/23) treatment is highly efficacious for psoriasis. Ustekinumab anti IL-12/23 antibody showed its efficacy and safety in three phase III trials recruiting 2899 patients. From two placebo controlled trials, PHOENIX 1 and PHOENIX 2, ustekinumab showed its efficacy in ameliorating psoriatic plaques, pruritus, and nail psoriasis [98]. (Table 1).

Remarkably, in a phase II multicenter, randomized, double-blind, placebo-controlled trial briakinumab, another human monoclonal anti-IL-12/23 antibody, 90-93% of subjects in 4 dosing groups were able to achieve a PASI 75 [99]. This finding alone confirms the centrality of this pathway because these levels of efficacy have not been previously seen in studies with other agents [100]. Safety data for both agents is limited, but to date has been favorable.

One issue with anti-p40 therapy is that it inhibits both the classical IL-12/Th1/IFN-γ and IL-23/Th17/IL-17 immune pathways. IL-12 and IL-23 are related cytokines with differences in their biological activities. After binding to their receptors, different intracellular transcription complexes are activated [101]. IL-12 predominantly acts on naïve T cells and initiates the TH1

PASI scores	Placebo [n = 410]	Ustekinumab (45 mg) [n = 409]	Ustekinumab (90 mg) [n = 411]
PASI 50	41 (10%)	342 (83.6%)*	367 (89.3%)*
PASI 75	15 (3.7%)	273 (66.7%)*	311 (75.7%)*
PASI 90	3 (0.7%)	173 (42.3%)*	209 (50.9%)*
Physician' s global assessment (Cleared)	0 (0.0%)	93 (22.7%)*	115 (28.0%)*
Physician' s global assessment (Cleared or minimal)	20 (4.9%)	278 (68%)*	302 (73.5%)*
Physician' s global assessment (marked or severe)	148 (36.1%)	15 (3.7%)*	10 (2.4%)*

* P <0.001 Adapted from: Papp KA, Langley RG, Lebwohl M, et al. Efficacy and safety of ustekinumab, a human interleukin-12/23 monoclonal antibody, in patients with psoriasis: 52-week results from a randomized, double-blind, placebo-controlled trial (PHOENIX 2) Lancet. 2008; 371(9625):1675-1684.

Table 1. Clinical improvement at week 12 (PHOENIX II)

response. In contrast, IL-23 primarily affects memory T cells and expands the initiated Th1 inflammatory response by Th17 activity and maintains an adequate memory pool by compromising memory T cells [64, 101, 102]. Experimental studies suggest that IL-23/Th17/IL-17 immune axis blocking is sufficient to treat autoimmune inflammation [63].

Another way to block both pathways is the immunoregulatory role of IFN-γ. It is well-known that the administration of anti-IFN-γ induces exacerbation of Experimental Autoimmune Encephalomyelitis (EAE) [103]. One possible explanation is the inhibition of IL-12/Th1/IFN-γ axis may destroy the regulatory role of IFN-γ during chronic inflammation. TNF-α, like INF-γ, has a regulatory role in the immune system [104]. This might explain the observation that anti-TNF therapies can induce psoriasis and other autoimmune diseases in some patients [105].

An increase in efficacy and reduction of adverse events are the main drivers for new therapies. Infections, one type of adverse event, usually increase in patients receiving anti-cytokine therapy [106]. Studies with anti-IL-23 therapy will require surveillance for the development of opportunistic infections. Reports from patients with IL-12 and/or IL-23 cytokine deficiency syndromes alert to these potential infections in individuals under anti-IL-23 therapy. Invasive salmonellosis and mycobacterial diseases were present more often in patients with IL-12/IL-23 deficiency indicating that immunity against these microorganisms appears to be dependent of IL-12 and/or IL-23 [107]. However, antibodies against IL-12 and IL-23 may not cause a complete inactivity of these cytokines in a clinical scenario. For example, an experimental study showed that IL-23 plays a role in host defense against *P. carinii*, but it is not an essential one [108]. Clinical studies with anti-IL-12/23 treatment thus far have not increased the risk of non opportunistic or opportunistic infections [109]. A recent study showed that blocking IL-23 with monoclonal antibodies during BCG infection does not appear to affect the bacterial burden in immunocompetent mice. In contrast, blocking TNF-α or both IL-23 and IL-12 with anti-p40 dramatically enhances mycobacterial growth. From this study, antibody blockade of IL-23 alone rather than IL-12 might be preferable in patients who have been, or may be, exposed to mycobacterial infection [110].

7. A new piece and a new move

As previously mentioned, the IL-23 favors the proliferation of the Th17 and consequent production of IL-22. IL-22 mRNA presence was initially described in IL-9 stimulated T-cell lines and in concanavalin A (Con-A)-activated murine spleen cells [111]. Further studies demonstrated that IL-22 expression can only be observed in activated immunological cells [112]. However, other reports have revealed that some T cells express IL-22 independently of IL-17 [113]. Finally, a new distinct human memory CD4+ T cell subset with skin-homing properties was identified and denominated Th22 [114].

A preferential production of IL-22 cytokine by T cells (Th22, Th17, and Th1) is present in psoriasis lesions [86]. Many animal models indicate the role of IL-22 in psoriasis. IL-22 over-expressed transgenic mice developed psoriasis-like skin lesions [115]. In IL-22 -/- mice, injection of IL-23 fails to induce epidermal hyperplasia indicating the role of IL-22 as a downstream mediator of tissue effects caused by IL-23 [78]. In a recent publication, Rizzo HL et al showed that to have IL-23 mediated epidermal hyperplasia, both IL-17 and IL-22 is required; any one of these is not sufficient to execute the effect of IL-23. They also showed that pre-treatment with anti IL-22 or anti IL-17A Abs block the rmIL-23 mediated epidermal hyperplasia in wild type mice [95]. In reconstituted epidermis model, IL-22 produces acanthosis dose dependently, which resembles psoriasis and either one of these alone is not sufficient to execute the effect of IL-23. The effects of IL-20 subfamily cytokines on reconstituted human epidermis suggest potential roles in cutaneous innate defense and pathogenic adaptive immunity in psoriasis [92]. In a study by Wolk K et al, a correlation was demonstrated between the plasma IL-22 levels and the severity of the disease [90]. IL-22 regulates the expression of genes responsible for antimicrobial defense, cellular differentiation, and mobility in keratinocytes and may play a: a potential role in psoriasis [90]. Moreover, IL-22 levels correlated with IL-20 levels, which is in accordance with the IL-22-induced keratinocyte IL-20 production [116]. This suggests that IL-22 and its downstream mediator IL-20 play an important role in the final steps of psoriasis pathogenesis. Sabat R and his group in their studies showed that IL-22 regulates keratinocyte function in several ways: a. IL-22 helps form a biological barrier of the skin by producing antimicrobial proteins (AMPs) like β-defensins, and S100 proteins. This may be one of the reasons that psoriatic patients have less skin infections. b. IL-22 interferes with physiological desquamation process of skin by inhibiting the terminal differentiation of keratinocytes. c. IL-22 plays a role in recruiting neutrophilic granulocytes in skin by inducing the production of chemokines;.

d. IL-22 indirectly helps in extracellular tissue degradation by inducing production of matrix metalloproteinases 1 and 3. IL-22 induces the production of IL-20, another IL-10 family cytokine which has similar effects as IL-22, thus resulting in amplification of the effects of IL-22 [117]. In a transgenic mouse model, it has been showed that IL-22 causes acanthosis, hyperkeratosis, and hypogranulosis, which are hallmarks of psoriasis. IL-22 acts through STAT-3 to impact the differentiation of keratinocytes [115]. IL-22 induces pro-inflammatory chemokines and antimicrobial proteins (AMPs) β-defensins (BDs), and promotes epidermal acanthosis and parakeratosis of keratinocytes [90, 118, 119]. Some synergistic effect was noted with other pro-inflammatory cytokines like TNF-α; IFN-γ; and IL-17 [117]. Alone, TNF- α does not have much effect on terminal differentiation of keratinocytes, but when keratinocytes were co-cultured with IL-22 and TNF- α, the effects of IL-22 were amplified. This kind of synergism was also seen with CXCL8 and IL-20 expression in keratinocytes co-stimulated with IL-22 & TNF-α. One possible explanation of this may be that TNF-α increases the expression of IL-22 receptor complex and also affects the IL-22 signaling pathway [115]. Thus, IL-22 and IL-20, but not IFN-γ or IL-17, are the key mediators of resulting epidermal proliferation. IL-22 acts through heterodimeric receptor complex composed of IL-22R1 and IL-10R2 [120]. IL-10R2 chain is ubiquitously expressed in all cells and is important component of receptor complexes required for IL-22, IL-10, IL-26 and IL-28 and IL-29, whereas the IL-22R1 chain is present in epithelial cells and hepatocytes [121]. Between the two subunits, IL-22 binds first to IL-22R1, the high-affinity receptor, and then IL-10R2, a lower affinity receptor [122]. To produce its effect, IL-22 acts through different signaling pathways, mainly signal transducer and activator of transcription 3 (STAT-3) and mitogen activated protein kinase [123].

This final move induces the vicious cycle of proliferation and inflammation of the skin characterized by the hyper-proliferative phenotype of keratinocytes in psoriasis. An anti-IL-22/IL-20 approach would have a complementary role to the neutralization of p40. However, there has not yet been a human study to demonstrate such a role or anti-IL-22 therapy in the treatment of psoriasis.

8. The other side of the chessboard: The role of T reg

Today, reading a book or scientific article on immunopathogensis, one will observe that suppressor T cells, renamed regulatory T cells (Tregs), have become a central concept in immunological vocabulary [124]. Hundreds of publications on Tregs have validated the existence of this single line of T cells. The CD4+CD25+highFoxp3+ Treg subpopulation is developed in the thymus and may be peripherally induced during the course of a normal immune response. The model in which Tregs directly or indirectly modify activation and differentiation of pathogenic T cells by means of an effect on antigen-presenting cells is supported by *in vivo* analyses [125].

8.1. Regulatory T cells: Development of an immunological concept

Biological systems are subject to complex regulatory controls and the immune system is no exception. It is known that the immune system has the potential to generate lymphocytes against auto-antigens. Experiments, however, suggest that individuals cannot easily be immunized against their own tissues. Therefore, a suppression mechanism is necessary to control potentially pathogenic immune cells. Owen suggested that this tolerance against one's own tissues is acquired during the development of the immune system, and Burnet proposed that the clonal selective destruction of lymphocytes for auto-antigens occurs primarily in the thymus.

The destruction of auto-reactive lymphocytes is the primary mechanism that leads to tolerance, but we know that this system is not perfect. Self-reactive B and T lymphocytes can be isolated from normal individuals [126]. Nishizuka and Sakakura proposed another mechanism for controlling auto-reactive cells. They observed that mice thymectomized between the second and fourth days of life developed an organ-specific autoimmune disease. This target-organ destruction can be prevented by restoring T cells from genetically identical individuals. The generation of regulator T cells was proposed in order to explain this mechanism of auto-tolerance attributed to the thymus [127].

Other studies observed that the prevention of autoimmune diseases was diminished by the reduction of CD4+ T cells, but not of CD8+ T cells, indicating that regulatory cells belonged to the CD4+ T cell class of lymphocytes. Sakaguchi subsequently characterized these regulatory cells as natural CD4+CD25+ Tregs that express Foxp3 [128].

8.2. Suppressor T cells: Regulatory T cells are suppressor T cells

Another control point of the immune response is established when the normal immune response is initiated. A different mechanism must be set off in order to control the magnitude of the response and its subsequent termination. This regulation should contribute to limiting clonal expansion and effector cell activity. Soon after the discovery that T lymphocytes function as helper cells for B-lymphocytes, RK Gershon proposed that they could also act as cells capable of suppressing the immune response [129]. This subpopulation of suppressor T cells was considered a controller of both auto-reactive and effector cells. A suppressor cell was functionally defined as a lymphocyte that inhibits the immune response by influencing the activity of another type of cell involved in a cascade of suppression factors, a network of anti-idiotypic T cells, and counter-suppressive cells [130].

Many of the experiments carried out contain data that support the existence of suppressor T cells. However, the mechanism responsible for these suppressive phenomena was never clearly characterized, and consequently interest in the field of suppressor T cells has gradually dwindled. The discovery of Th1/Th2 cells led researchers to abandon the concept of suppressor T cells. Suppression was instead attributed to counter-regulatory cytokines. As pointed out by Green and Webb, the letter "S" started to resemble a foul word in cellular immunology, and its use was considered synonymous of scarce data with excessive interpretation or a mystic phenomenon [131].

http://dx.doi.org/10.5772/53580

Suppressor T cells reappeared as regulatory T cells (Tregs) in the late 1990s when several subpopulations of T cells were identified as having the capacity to inhibit the proliferation of other cells. Shevach et al. were the first to call attention to the fact that regulatory T cells and suppressor T cells are the same [132]. Therefore, the term 'regulatory' gradually replaced the term 'suppressor'. The main problem, however, is not that cells are termed regulatory, but that they are considered to be suppressors. It is more appropriate to consider regulatory T cells as immune response directors instead of its suppressors.

9. Regulatory T cells and psoriasis

The regulation mechanism of the immune system by CD25+high Tregs is not well understood. Studies have not yet arrived at a simple mode of action. Whatever the mechanism, the homeostatic balance of the immune system is obtained by healthy cellular and humoral responses. Some inflammatory agents, whether physical, chemical, or infectious, induce an intense immune response. This immune response against them frequently results in tissue damage that could be more intense if it were not for the interference of regulatory mechanisms [133]. As has already been specified, Treg cells help limit the damage caused by a vigorous immune response. Natural Treg cells may respond to an ample variety of auto-antigens, although there is evidence that they may also respond to antigens expressed by microbes. Induced regulatory T cells, such as TR1 or Th3, may develop from CD4+ T cells when exposed to specific conditions [134].

Similarly, excessive activity of Treg cells may limit the magnitude of the immune response, which may result in failure to control an infection. On the other hand, the absence of the T regulator may result in intense inflammation and autoimmune dermatitis. Tissue damage may also result from the development of effector cells against their own auto-antigens (Figure 4).

Psoriasis is sustained by the activation of pathogenic T cells. The regulatory expression of skin diseases discusses the action exerted by regulatory T cells, especially CD4+CD25+high Tregs on psoriasis. Various types of influence of these cells suggest that they may act by suppressing or augmenting immunity [135, 136]. The control of Treg cells may affect the results favorably or may be deleterious. There is no definitive view. In psoriasis, studies have shown that the subpopulation of CD4+ T lymphocytes in peripheral blood, phenotypically CD25+high, CTLA-4(+), Foxp3high, is deficient in its suppressor functions. This is associated with an accelerated proliferation of the CD4+ T cell response [137]. The presence of non-functional CD4+CD25+high Treg cells in peripheral blood and in tissues may lead to a reduced capacity to contain pathogenic T cells and to a hyperproliferation of the psoriatic plaque *in vivo*. These findings represent a critical component of this autoimmune disease and may have implications for potential therapy by manipulation of CD4+CD25+high Tregs *in vivo*. However, other factors, such as the immune status and genotype, and the presence of concomitant diseases or other infections may also have an influence. The manipulation of this balance can be explored therapeutically.

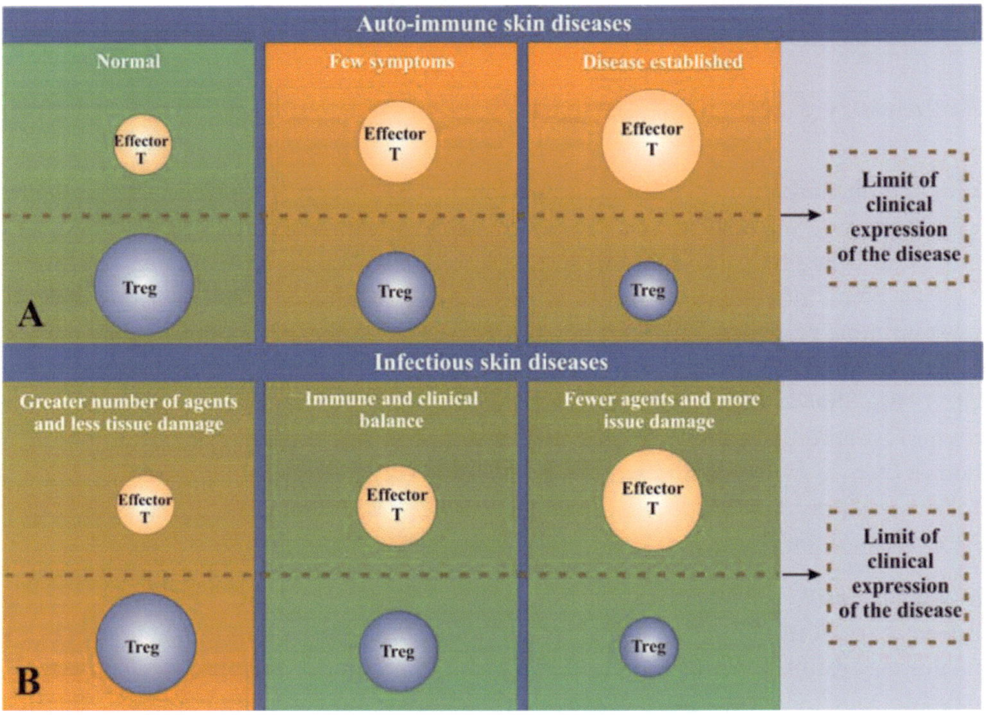

Figure 4. Immune response regulation mechanisms. The force balance between Tregs and the effector T CD4+ cells may present in a different manner depending on being an autoantigen or a pathogen. In A portion, the clinical expression of autoimmune skin diseases is shown. In this case, there is clinical manifestation only when the number and function of Tregs are significantly reduced. B portion displays clinical manifestations that may occur in extreme cases. In case of excessive Treg function, the result shows reduction of effector lymphocytes against the pathogen, an increase in its number and less tissue damage. The contrary applies to effector cells against the pathogen that surpass the number and function of Treg. The ideal immune and clinical response occurs when there is a balance between functions

9.1. Clinical and therapeutic consequences of regulatory T cells

An improved understanding of the role of T regulators in psoriasis may lead to the identification of new targets for treatment. More specifically, the goal is to manipulate natural regulator cells or those induced by means of an increase or decrease of their function, depending on the circumstances.

Auto-injections of regulatory T cells are a promising approach to modulation of inflammation and autoimmune diseases [138]. Nevertheless, there is a significant decline in the function of natural CD4+CD25+high Treg cells of peripheral blood in patients with autoimmune diseases when compared to that of healthy individuals. In order to overcome this difficulty, cytokines were used to stimulate the growth of regulator T cells. IL-15 allows a significant *in vitro* expansion of regulator cells [139]. Natural CD4+CD25+high Treg cells obtained by *ex vivo* expansion through stimulation with allogeneic antigen-presenting cells and IL-2 were capable of modulating the graft-versus-host disease (GVHD). Induction of natural CD4+CD25+high Treg cells may facilitate the establishment and maintenance of immunological tolerance. Depletion of natural CD4+CD25+high Treg cells may be an effective way of reversing the tolerance induced by malignant tumors and increasing the activity of the immune system against cancer epitopes [140].

In the field of dermatology, the stimulation of Treg cells may be important in autoimmune diseases. For example, blockage of T lymphocyte stimulation, as in the use of the antibody associated with CTLA-4 (cytotoxic T lymphocyte-associated antigen 4-immunoglobulin, CTLA4Ig), reverts the development of psoriatic plaques [141]. In the clinical context, the effect of immunomodulator drugs on these cells warrants attention. For example, tacrolimus, an inhibitor of calcineurin, increases the inhibition of Treg cells in atopic dermatitis [142, 143]. Fludarabine reduces the frequency and suppressive function of natural CD4+CD25+high Treg cells [144]. Low doses of cyclophosphamide induce the inhibition of natural CD4+CD25+high Treg cells and consequently increase the immune response in an apparently paradoxical effect [145]. Along the same line, cyclophosphamide decreases the function, proportion, and number of natural CD4+CD25+high Treg cells that suppress the induction of contact hypersensitivity [146, 147]. Currently, topical corticosteroids constitute one of the most effective treatments for psoriasis and other inflammatory skin diseases. These drugs are effective in inhibiting the function of Th2 cells, eosinophils, and epithelial cells. However, treatment with these drugs during the presentation of the epitope may result in an increased tolerance by suppressing the development of dendrite cells that secrete IL-10, which are necessary for the induction of T regulators. Therefore, treatment with corticosteroids may increase the subsequent effect of the T response and aggravate, on the long run, the course of inflammatory diseases [148]. This aspect may also be related to the rebound effect of inflammatory diseases once these drugs are removed.

10. What is new?

Studies suggest that IL-23/Th17/IL-17 immune axis blocking can be used to treat psoriasis [63]. Ustekinumab, anti IL-12/23 antibody, showed its efficacy in ameliorating psoriatic plaques, pruritus, and nail psoriasis [98]. This stimulated growing interest in the therapeutic potential of agents such as brodalumab, ixekizumab, and secukinumab that inhibit interleukin-17 signaling. These new group of biologics are in clinical trials. They use cytokine neutralization and receptor antagonism in treating psoriasis. Secukinumab and ixekizumab specifically neutralize interleukin-17A, whereas brodalumab is an antagonist of the interleukin-17RA receptor [149-151].

As previously mentioned, IL-23 favors the proliferation of the Th17 and consequent production of IL-22. Fezakinumab (ILV-094, Pfizer) is a fully human monoclonal IgGγ antibody to IL-22 under study for the treatment of rheumatoid arthritis and psoriasis [152].

Nonetheless, there is no single new data about the basic mechanisms of psoriasis development despite the cytokine and anti-cytokine therapies widely used.

11. Conclusion

In medicine, a gold standard is the intervention believed to be the best available option. Given the proven role of many cytokines in psoriasis, substantial interest exists in targeting them with neutralization immunotherapy. If Th1/Th17/Th22 pathways operate in different steps of psoriasis development, then targeted blockade place biologics as the standard-setting paradigm for therapy and understanding of the pathogenesis of psoriasis. However, large studies are needed to provide information on the therapeutic effects, adverse events of any anti-cytokine therapy, and their place in the treatment of psoriasis and other skin diseases. To complement this approach, a detailed comprehension of the associations among the various regulator cells may help in understanding the events leading to the genesis of skin diseases. Ultimately, an ability to manipulate the function of regulator T cells according to the desired therapeutic effect will be the goal. Together, an integrated immunologic approach to therapy holds great promise in reducing the burden of psoriatic disease.

Now that cytokine and anti-cytokine therapies are increasingly used, it is a great opportunity to learn in detail the complex action of these molecules, including both their pro-inflammatory and immunosuppressive properties. The data present above clearly indicate that autoimmunity is a complex system. The immune response seems to be in a constant balancing act with itself. Emerging data indicate that a more realistic view is that these cytokines are not especially loyal to their functions. They switch sides, meaning that they do not have simple pro- or anti-inflammatory actions.

Therefore, the mechanisms of action of the biologic therapies are more intricate than a simple blocking effect. The same cytokine can promote immune and inflammatory responses in some circumstances and inhibit responses in other settings. There is good and bad in every cytokine. Finally, the gut, skin or oral microbial communities simply primes the immune system. Therefore, psoriasis is a game played by many pieces and movements on a complex chessboard. The combinations of movements (cytokines) exert variable effects at different times during the evolution of autoimmune disease. There is much left to be done to dissect the complex and highly interactive effects of the players that one would have thought we understood very well, the Immunology game's inner logic. The application of game theory to Immunology thinking is our new proposition to explain autoimmune diseases and other immunologic responses. The objective is taking game theory seriously as a potential source of insight into the complex relationships that determine immune system function.

Author details

Robyn S Fallen[1], Anupam Mitra[2], Laura Morrisey[1] and Hermenio Lima[3*]

*Address all correspondence to: hlima@mcmaster.ca

1 Michael G. DeGroote School of Medicine - Waterloo Regional Campus - McMaster University, Canada

2 UC Davis School of Medicine, Allergy and Clinical Immunology, Mather, CA, USA

3 Division of Dermatology, Department of Medicine, Michael G. DeGroote School of Medicine, McMaster University, Canada

References

[1] Vaz, N. M, Ramos, G. C, Pordeus, V, & Carvalho, C. R. The conservative physiology of the immune system. A non-metaphoric approach to immunological activity. Clin Dev Immunol. (2006). Jun-Dec;13(2-4):133-42.

[2] Scarpa, R, Altomare, G, Marchesoni, A, & Balato, N. Matucci Cerinic M, Lotti T, et al. Psoriatic disease: concepts and implications. J Eur Acad Dermatol Venereol. (2010). Jun;, 24(6), 627-30.

[3] Lima, X. T, Seidler, E. M, Lima, H. C, & Kimball, A. B. Long-term safety of biologics in dermatology. Dermatol Ther. (2009). Jan-Feb;, 22(1), 2-21.

[4] Feldmann, M, Brennan, F. M, & Maini, R. Cytokines in autoimmune disorders. Int Rev Immunol. (1998).

[5] Squire, B. The Etiology of Psoriasis. Br Med J. (1873). Feb):141.

[6] Heaney, J. H. The Etiology and Treatment of Psoriasis. Br Med J. (1927). Dec):, 1136-7.

[7] Ingram, J. T. The approach to psoriasis. Br Med J. (1953). Sep 12;, 2(4836), 591-4.

[8] Harber, L. C, March, C, & Ovary, Z. Lack of passive cutaneous anaphylaxis in psoriasis. Arch Dermatol. (1962). Jun;, 85, 716-9.

[9] Aswaq, M, Farber, E. M, Moreci, A. P, & Raffel, S. Immunologic reactions in psoriasis. Arch Dermatol. (1960). Nov;, 82, 663-6.

[10] Landau, J, Gross, B. G, Newcomer, V. D, & Wright, E. T. Immunologic Response of Patients with Psoriasis. Arch Dermatol. (1965). Jun;, 91, 607-10.

[11] Harris, C. C. Malignancy during methotrexate and steroid therapy for psoriasis. Arch Dermatol. (1971). May;, 103(5), 501-4.

[12] Shuster, S. Research into psoriasis--the last decade. Br Med J. (1971). Jul 24;, 3(5768), 236-9.

[13] Hunter, J. A, Ryan, T. J, & Savin, J. A. Diseases of the skin. Present and future trends in approaches to skin disease. Br Med J. (1974). Feb 16;, 1(5902), 283-4.

[14] Braun-falco, O, & Christophers, E. Structural aspects of initial psoriatic lesions. Arch Dermatol Forsch. (1974)., 251(2), 95-110.

[15] Krueger, G. G, Jederberg, W. W, Ogden, B. E, & Reese, D. L. Inflammatory and immune cell function in psoriasis: II. Monocyte function, lymphokine production. J Invest Dermatol. (1978). Sep;, 71(3), 195-201.

[16] Krueger, G. G, & Jederberg, W. W. Alteration of HeLa cell growth equilibrium by supernatants of peripheral blood mononuclear cells from normal and psoriatic subjects. J Invest Dermatol. (1980). Mar;, 74(3), 148-53.

[17] Champion, R. H. Psoriasis and its treatment. Br Med J (Clin Res Ed). (1981). Jan 31;, 282(6261), 343-6.

[18] Bos, J. D, Hulsebosch, H. J, Krieg, S. R, Bakker, P. M, & Cormane, R. H. Immunocompetent cells in psoriasis. In situ immunophenotyping by monoclonal antibodies. Arch Dermatol Res. (1983)., 275(3), 181-9.

[19] Baker, B. S, Swain, A. F, Griffiths, C. E, Leonard, J. N, Fry, L, & Valdimarsson, H. The effects of topical treatment with steroids or dithranol on epidermal T lymphocytes and dendritic cells in psoriasis. Scand J Immunol. (1985). Nov;, 22(5), 471-7.

[20] Bos, J. D, & Krieg, S. R. Psoriasis infiltrating cell immunophenotype: changes induced by PUVA or corticosteroid treatment in T-cell subsets, Langerhans' cells and interdigitating cells. Acta Derm Venereol. (1985)., 65(5), 390-7.

[21] Lieden, G, & Skogh, M. Plasma exchange and leukapheresis in psoriasis--no effect? Arch Dermatol Res. (1986)., 278(6), 437-40.

[22] Valdimarsson, H, Bake, B. S, Jónsdótdr, I, & Fry, L. Psoriasis: a disease of abnormal Keratinocyte proliferation induced by T lymphocytes. Immunology Today. (1986)., 7(9), 256-9.

[23] Schlaak, J. F, Buslau, M, Jochum, W, Hermann, E, Girndt, M, Gallati, H, et al. T cells involved in psoriasis vulgaris belong to the Th1 subset. J Invest Dermatol. (1994). Feb;, 102(2), 145-9.

[24] Mosmann, T. R, Cherwinski, H, Bond, M. W, Giedlin, M. A, & Coffman, R. L. Two types of murine helper T cell clone. I. Definition according to profiles of lymphokine activities and secreted proteins. J Immunol. (1986). Apr 1;, 136(7), 2348-57.

[25] Austin, L. M, Ozawa, M, Kikuchi, T, Walters, I. B, & Krueger, J. G. The majority of epidermal T cells in Psoriasis vulgaris lesions can produce type 1 cytokines, interferon-gamma, interleukin-2, and tumor necrosis factor-alpha, defining TC1 (cytotoxic T

lymphocyte) and TH1 effector populations: a type 1 differentiation bias is also measured in circulating blood T cells in psoriatic patients. J Invest Dermatol. (1999). Nov;, 113(5), 752-9.

[26] Kagami, S, Rizzo, H. L, Kurtz, S. E, Miller, L. S, Blauvelt, A, But, I. L-23 a. n. d I. L-17A, & Not, I. L. and IL-22, are required for optimal skin host defense against Candida albicans. J Immunol. (2010). Nov 1;, 185(9), 5453-62.

[27] Abdi, K. IL-12: the role of versus p75. Scand J Immunol. (2002). Jul;56(1):1-11., 40.

[28] Vanaudenaerde, B. M, Verleden, S. E, Vos, R, De Vleeschauwer, S. I, Willems-widyastuti, A, Geenens, R, et al. Innate and Adaptive IL-17 Producing Lymphocytes in Chronic Inflammatory Lung Disorders. Am J Respir Crit Care Med. (2010). Nov 19.

[29] Nickoloff, B. J, & Nestle, F. O. Recent insights into the immunopathogenesis of psoriasis provide new therapeutic opportunities. J Clin Invest. (2004). Jun;, 113(12), 1664-75.

[30] Kraan, M. C, Van Kuijk, A. W, Dinant, H. J, Goedkoop, A. Y, Smeets, T. J, De Rie, M. A, et al. Alefacept treatment in psoriatic arthritis: reduction of the effector T cell population in peripheral blood and synovial tissue is associated with improvement of clinical signs of arthritis. Arthritis Rheum. (2002). Oct;, 46(10), 2776-84.

[31] Kalliolias, G. D, Gordon, R. A, & Ivashkiv, L. B. Suppression of TNF-alpha and IL-1 signaling identifies a mechanism of homeostatic regulation of macrophages by IL-27. J Immunol. (2010). Dec 1;, 185(11), 7047-56.

[32] Philipp, S, Wolk, K, Kreutzer, S, Wallace, E, Ludwig, N, Roewert, J, et al. The evaluation of psoriasis therapy with biologics leads to a revision of the current view of the pathogenesis of this disorder. Expert Opin Ther Targets. (2006). Dec;, 10(6), 817-31.

[33] Sobell, J. M, Kalb, R. E, & Weinberg, J. M. Management of moderate to severe plaque psoriasis (part 2): clinical update on T-cell modulators and investigational agents. J Drugs Dermatol. (2009). Mar;, 8(3), 230-8.

[34] Monteleone, G, & Pallone, F. MacDonald TT, Chimenti S, Costanzo A. Psoriasis: from pathogenesis to novel therapeutic approaches. Clin Sci (Lond). (2011). Jan;, 120(1), 1-11.

[35] Albanesi, C, & Pastore, S. Pathobiology of chronic inflammatory skin diseases: interplay between keratinocytes and immune cells as a target for anti-inflammatory drugs. Curr Drug Metab. (2010). Mar;, 11(3), 210-27.

[36] Endo, Y, Tamura, A, Ishikawa, O, Miyachi, Y, & Hashimoto, T. Psoriasis vulgaris coexistent with epidermolysis bullosa acquisita. Br J Dermatol. (1997). Nov;, 137(5), 783-6.

[37] Albanesi, C, De Pita, O, & Girolomoni, G. Resident skin cells in psoriasis: a special look at the pathogenetic functions of keratinocytes. Clin Dermatol. (2007). Nov-Dec;, 25(6), 581-8.

[38] Chen, S. C, De Groot, M, Kinsley, D, Laverty, M, Mcclanahan, T, Arreaza, M, et al. Expression of chemokine receptor CXCR3 by lymphocytes and plasmacytoid dendritic cells in human psoriatic lesions. Arch Dermatol Res. (2010). Mar;, 302(2), 113-23.

[39] Lima Ede ALima Mde A. Reviewing concepts in the immunopathogenesis of psoriasis. An Bras Dermatol. (2011). Nov-Dec;, 86(6), 1151-8.

[40] Krishnamurthy, K, Walker, A, Gropper, C. A, & Hoffman, C. To treat or not to treat? Management of guttate psoriasis and pityriasis rosea in patients with evidence of group A Streptococcal infection. J Drugs Dermatol. (2010). Mar;, 9(3), 241-50.

[41] Bangert, C, Brunner, P. M, & Stingl, G. Immune functions of the skin. Clin Dermatol. (2011). Jul-Aug;, 29(4), 360-76.

[42] Sercarz, E, & Maverakis, E. van den Elzen P, Madakamutil L, Kumar V. Seven surprises in the TCR-centred regulation of immune responsiveness in an autoimmune system. Novartis Found Symp. (2003). discussion 71-6, 203-10., 252, 165-71.

[43] Iversen, O. J, Lysvand, H, & Hagen, L. The autoantigen Pso a post-translational modification of SCCA molecules. Autoimmunity. (2011). May;44(3):229-34., 27.

[44] Kaufmann, S. H. Elie Metchnikoff's and Paul Ehrlich's impact on infection biology. Microbes Infect. (2008). Nov-Dec;10(14-15):1417-9.

[45] Von Neumann, J, & Morgenstern, O. Theory of games and economic behavior. Princeton: Princeton university press; (1944).

[46] Gewin, V. The skin's secret surveillance system. Nature Publishing Group; (2012). updated Jul 26, 2012; cited 2012 September 2, 2012]; Available from: http://www.nature.com/news/the-skin-s-secret-surveillance-system-1.11075.

[47] Naik, S, Bouladoux, N, Wilhelm, C, Molloy, M. J, Salcedo, R, Kastenmuller, W, et al. Compartmentalized control of skin immunity by resident commensals. Science. (2012). Aug 31;, 337(6098), 1115-9.

[48] Morizane, S, & Gallo, R. L. Antimicrobial peptides in the pathogenesis of psoriasis. J Dermatol. (2012). Mar;, 39(3), 225-30.

[49] Fung, I, Garrett, J. P, Shahane, A, & Kwan, M. Do Bugs Control Our Fate? The Influence of the Microbiome on Autoimmunity. Curr Allergy Asthma Rep. (2012). Aug 11.

[50] Smith, J. M. The theory of games and the evolution of animal conflicts. J Theor Biol. (1974). Sep;, 47(1), 209-21.

[51] Steinbeck, J, & Astro, R. The Log from the Sea of Cortez: Penguin Books Limited; (2001).

[52] Rook, G. A. Hygiene hypothesis and autoimmune diseases. Clin Rev Allergy Immunol. (2012). Feb;, 42(1), 5-15.

[53] Albanesi, C, Scarponi, C, Giustizieri, M. L, & Girolomoni, G. Keratinocytes in inflammatory skin diseases. Curr Drug Targets Inflamm Allergy. (2005). Jun;, 4(3), 329-34.

[54] Lowes, M. A, Bowcock, A. M, & Krueger, J. G. Pathogenesis and therapy of psoriasis. Nature. (2007). Feb 22;, 445(7130), 866-73.

[55] Schon, M. P, & Boehncke, W. H. Psoriasis. N Engl J Med. (2005). May 5;, 352(18), 1899-912.

[56] Nickoloff, B. J, & Schroder, J. M. von den Driesch P, Raychaudhuri SP, Farber EM, Boehncke WH, et al. Is psoriasis a T-cell disease? Exp Dermatol. (2000). Oct;, 9(5), 359-75.

[57] Okamura, H, Tsutsi, H, Komatsu, T, Yutsudo, M, Hakura, A, Tanimoto, T, et al. Cloning of a new cytokine that induces IFN-gamma production by T cells. Nature. (1995). Nov 2;, 378(6552), 88-91.

[58] Biedermann, T, Rocken, M, & Carballido, J. M. TH1 and TH2 lymphocyte development and regulation of TH cell-mediated immune responses of the skin. J Investig Dermatol Symp Proc. (2004). Jan;, 9(1), 5-14.

[59] Macatonia, S. E, Hosken, N. A, Litton, M, Vieira, P, Hsieh, C. S, Culpepper, J. A, et al. Dendritic cells produce IL-12 and direct the development of Th1 cells from naive CD4+ T cells. J Immunol. (1995). May 15;, 154(10), 5071-9.

[60] Trinchieri, G. Interleukin-12: a cytokine at the interface of inflammation and immunity. Adv Immunol. (1998)., 70, 83-243.

[61] Hong, K, Berg, E. L, & Ehrhardt, R. O. Persistence of pathogenic CD4+ Th1-like cells in vivo in the absence of IL-12 but in the presence of autoantigen. J Immunol. (2001). Apr 1;, 166(7), 4765-72.

[62] Hong, K, Chu, A, Ludviksson, B. R, Berg, E. L, & Ehrhardt, R. O. IL-12, independently of IFN-gamma, plays a crucial role in the pathogenesis of a murine psoriasis-like skin disorder. J Immunol. (1999). Jun 15;, 162(12), 7480-91.

[63] Monteleone, I, Pallone, F, & Monteleone, G. Interleukin-23 and Th17 cells in the control of gut inflammation. Mediators Inflamm. (2009).

[64] Oppmann, B, Lesley, R, Blom, B, Timans, J. C, Xu, Y, Hunte, B, et al. Novel protein engages IL-12p40 to form a cytokine, IL-23, with biological activities similar as well as distinct from IL-12. Immunity. (2000). Nov;13(5):715-25., 19.

[65] Lee, E, Trepicchio, W. L, Oestreicher, J. L, Pittman, D, Wang, F, Chamian, F, et al. Increased expression of interleukin 23 and p40 in lesional skin of patients with psoriasis vulgaris. J Exp Med. (2004). Jan 5;199(1):125-30., 19.

[66] Toichi, E, Torres, G, Mccormick, T. S, Chang, T, Mascelli, M. A, Kauffman, C. L, et al. An anti-IL-12antibody down-regulates type 1 cytokines, chemokines, and IL-12/IL-23 in psoriasis. J Immunol. (2006). Oct 1;177(7):4917-26., 40.

[67] Piskin, G, Sylva-steenland, R. M, Bos, J. D, & Teunissen, M. B. In vitro and in situ expression of IL-23 by keratinocytes in healthy skin and psoriasis lesions: enhanced expression in psoriatic skin. J Immunol. (2006). Feb 1;, 176(3), 1908-15.

[68] Wilson, N. J, Boniface, K, Chan, J. R, Mckenzie, B. S, Blumenschein, W. M, Mattson, J. D, et al. Development, cytokine profile and function of human interleukin 17-producing helper T cells. Nat Immunol. (2007). Sep;, 8(9), 950-7.

[69] Lillis, J. V, Guo, C. S, Lee, J. J, Blauvelt, A, & Increased, I. L. expression in palmoplantar psoriasis and hyperkeratotic hand dermatitis. Arch Dermatol. (2010). Aug;, 146(8), 918-9.

[70] Capon, F. Di Meglio P, Szaub J, Prescott NJ, Dunster C, Baumber L, et al. Sequence variants in the genes for the interleukin-23 receptor (IL23R) and its ligand (IL12B) confer protection against psoriasis. Hum Genet. (2007). Sep;, 122(2), 201-6.

[71] Cargill, M, Schrodi, S. J, Chang, M, Garcia, V. E, Brandon, R, Callis, K. P, et al. A large-scale genetic association study confirms IL12B and leads to the identification of IL23R as psoriasis-risk genes. Am J Hum Genet. (2007). Feb;, 80(2), 273-90.

[72] Nair, R. P, Ding, J, Duffin, K. C, Helms, C, Voorhees, J. J, Krueger, G. G, et al. Psoriasis bench to bedside: genetics meets immunology. Arch Dermatol. (2009). Apr;, 145(4), 462-4.

[73] Tonel, G, Conrad, C, & Laggner, U. Di Meglio P, Grys K, McClanahan TK, et al. Cutting edge: A critical functional role for IL-23 in psoriasis. J Immunol. (2010). Nov 15;, 185(10), 5688-91.

[74] Aggarwal, S, Ghilardi, N, Xie, M. H, De Sauvage, F. J, & Gurney, A. L. Interleukin-23 promotes a distinct CD4 T cell activation state characterized by the production of interleukin-17. J Biol Chem. (2003). Jan 17;, 278(3), 1910-4.

[75] Miossec, P, Korn, T, & Kuchroo, V. K. Interleukin-17 and type 17 helper T cells. N Engl J Med. (2009). Aug 27;, 361(9), 888-98.

[76] Romagnani, S, Maggi, E, Liotta, F, Cosmi, L, & Annunziato, F. Properties and origin of human Th17 cells. Mol Immunol. (2009). Nov;, 47(1), 3-7.

[77] Korn, T, Bettelli, E, Oukka, M, Kuchroo, V. K, & Th, I. L. Cells. Annu Rev Immunol. (2009)., 27, 485-517.

[78] Zheng, Y, Danilenko, D. M, Valdez, P, Kasman, I, Eastham-anderson, J, Wu, J, et al. Interleukin-22, a T(H)17 cytokine, mediates IL-23-induced dermal inflammation and acanthosis. Nature. (2007). Feb 8;, 445(7128), 648-51.

[79] Ghoreschi, K, Laurence, A, Yang, X. P, Tato, C. M, Mcgeachy, M. J, Konkel, J. E, et al. Generation of pathogenic T(H)17 cells in the absence of TGF-beta signalling. Nature. (2010). Oct 21;, 467(7318), 967-71.

[80] Volpe, E, Servant, N, Zollinger, R, Bogiatzi, S. I, Hupe, P, Barillot, E, et al. A critical function for transforming growth factor-beta, interleukin 23 and proinflammatory cytokines in driving and modulating human T(H)-17 responses. Nat Immunol. (2008). Jun;, 9(6), 650-7.

[81] Infante-duarte, C, Horton, H. F, Byrne, M. C, & Kamradt, T. Microbial lipopeptides induce the production of IL-17 in Th cells. J Immunol. (2000). Dec 1;, 165(11), 6107-15.

[82] Harrington, L. E, Hatton, R. D, Mangan, P. R, Turner, H, Murphy, T. L, Murphy, K. M, et al. Interleukin 17-producing CD4+ effector T cells develop via a lineage distinct from the T helper type 1 and 2 lineages. Nat Immunol. (2005). Nov;, 6(11), 1123-32.

[83] Zaba, L. C, Cardinale, I, Gilleaudeau, P, Sullivan-whalen, M, Suarez-farinas, M, Fuentes-duculan, J, et al. Amelioration of epidermal hyperplasia by TNF inhibition is associated with reduced Th17 responses. J Exp Med. (2007). Dec 24;, 204(13), 3183-94.

[84] Harper, E. G, Guo, C, Rizzo, H, Lillis, J. V, Kurtz, S. E, Skorcheva, I, et al. Th17 cytokines stimulate CCL20 expression in keratinocytes in vitro and in vivo: implications for psoriasis pathogenesis. J Invest Dermatol. (2009). Sep;, 129(9), 2175-83.

[85] Johansen, C, Usher, P. A, Kjellerup, R. B, Lundsgaard, D, Iversen, L, & Kragballe, K. Characterization of the interleukin-17 isoforms and receptors in lesional psoriatic skin. Br J Dermatol. (2009). Feb;, 160(2), 319-24.

[86] Lowes, M. A, Kikuchi, T, Fuentes-duculan, J, Cardinale, I, Zaba, L. C, Haider, A. S, et al. Psoriasis vulgaris lesions contain discrete populations of Th1 and Th17 T cells. J Invest Dermatol. (2008). May;, 128(5), 1207-11.

[87] Boniface, K, Guignouard, E, Pedretti, N, Garcia, M, Delwail, A, Bernard, F. X, et al. A role for T cell-derived interleukin 22 in psoriatic skin inflammation. Clin Exp Immunol. (2007). Dec;, 150(3), 407-15.

[88] Nograles, K. E, Zaba, L. C, Guttman-yassky, E, Fuentes-duculan, J, Suarez-farinas, M, Cardinale, I, et al. Th17 cytokines interleukin (IL)-17 and IL-22 modulate distinct inflammatory and keratinocyte-response pathways. Br J Dermatol. (2008). Nov;, 159(5), 1092-102.

[89] Albanesi, C, Scarponi, C, Cavani, A, Federici, M, Nasorri, F, & Girolomoni, G. Interleukin-17 is produced by both Th1 and Th2 lymphocytes, and modulates interferon-gamma- and interleukin-4-induced activation of human keratinocytes. J Invest Dermatol. (2000). Jul;, 115(1), 81-7.

[90] Wolk, K, Witte, E, Wallace, E, Docke, W. D, Kunz, S, Asadullah, K, et al. IL-22 regulates the expression of genes responsible for antimicrobial defense, cellular differentiation, and mobility in keratinocytes: a potential role in psoriasis. Eur J Immunol. (2006). May;, 36(5), 1309-23.

[91] Liang, S. C, Tan, X. Y, Luxenberg, D. P, Karim, R, Dunussi-joannopoulos, K, Collins, M, et al. Interleukin (IL)-22 and IL-17 are coexpressed by Th17 cells and cooperatively enhance expression of antimicrobial peptides. J Exp Med. (2006). Oct 2;, 203(10), 2271-9.

[92] Sa, S. M, Valdez, P. A, Wu, J, Jung, K, Zhong, F, Hall, L, et al. The effects of IL-20 subfamily cytokines on reconstituted human epidermis suggest potential roles in cutaneous innate defense and pathogenic adaptive immunity in psoriasis. J Immunol. (2007). Feb 15;, 178(4), 2229-40.

[93] Chan, J. R, Blumenschein, W, Murphy, E, Diveu, C, Wiekowski, M, Abbondanzo, S, et al. IL-23 stimulates epidermal hyperplasia via TNF and IL-20R2-dependent mechanisms with implications for psoriasis pathogenesis. J Exp Med. (2006). Nov 27;, 203(12), 2577-87.

[94] Kopp, T, Lenz, P, Bello-fernandez, C, Kastelein, R. A, Kupper, T. S, & Stingl, G. IL-23 production by cosecretion of endogenous and transgenic p40 in keratin 14/p40 transgenic mice: evidence for enhanced cutaneous immunity. J Immunol. (2003). Jun 1;170(11):5438-44., 19.

[95] Rizzo, H. L, Kagami, S, Phillips, K. G, Kurtz, S. E, Jacques, S. L, Blauvelt, A, & Psoriasis-like, I. L-23-m. e. d. i. a. t. e. d. epidermal hyperplasia is dependent on IL-17A. J Immunol. (2011). Feb 1;, 186(3), 1495-502.

[96] Nestle, F. O, Kaplan, D. H, & Barker, J. Psoriasis. N Engl J Med. (2009). Jul 30;, 361(5), 496-509.

[97] Watanabe, H, Kawaguchi, M, Fujishima, S, Ogura, M, Matsukura, S, Takeuchi, H, et al. Functional characterization of IL-17F as a selective neutrophil attractant in psoriasis. J Invest Dermatol. (2009). Mar;, 129(3), 650-6.

[98] Yeilding, N, Szapary, P, Brodmerkel, C, Benson, J, Plotnick, M, Zhou, H, et al. Development of the IL-12/23 antagonist ustekinumab in psoriasis: past, present, and future perspectives. Ann N Y Acad Sci. (2011). Mar;, 1222, 30-9.

[99] Lima, X. T, Abuabara, K, Kimball, A. B, & Lima, H. C. Briakinumab. Expert Opin Biol Ther. (2009). Aug;, 9(8), 1107-13.

[100] Leonardi, C. L, Kimball, A. B, Papp, K. A, Yeilding, N, Guzzo, C, Wang, Y, et al. Efficacy and safety of ustekinumab, a human interleukin-12/23 monoclonal antibody, in patients with psoriasis: 76-week results from a randomised, double-blind, placebo-controlled trial (PHOENIX 1). Lancet. (2008). May 17;, 371(9625), 1665-74.

[101] Parham, C, Chirica, M, Timans, J, Vaisberg, E, Travis, M, Cheung, J, et al. A receptor for the heterodimeric cytokine IL-23 is composed of IL-12Rbeta1 and a novel cytokine receptor subunit, IL-23R. J Immunol. (2002). Jun 1;, 168(11), 5699-708.

[102] Trinchieri, G, Pflanz, S, Kastelein, R. A, & The, I. L. family of heterodimeric cytokines: new players in the regulation of T cell responses. Immunity. (2003). Nov;, 19(5), 641-4.

[103] Becher, B, Durell, B. G, & Noelle, R. J. Experimental autoimmune encephalitis and inflammation in the absence of interleukin-12. J Clin Invest. (2002). Aug;, 110(4), 493-7.

[104] Liu, J, Marino, M. W, Wong, G, Grail, D, Dunn, A, Bettadapura, J, et al. TNF is a potent anti-inflammatory cytokine in autoimmune-mediated demyelination. Nat Med. (1998). Jan;, 4(1), 78-83.

[105] Ramos-casals, M, Brito-zeron, P, Soto, M. J, Cuadrado, M. J, & Khamashta, M. A. Autoimmune diseases induced by TNF-targeted therapies. Best Pract Res Clin Rheumatol. (2008). Oct;, 22(5), 847-61.

[106] Dinarello, C. A. Anti-cytokine therapeutics and infections. Vaccine. (2003). Jun 1;21 Suppl 2:S, 24-34.

[107] MacLennan CFieschi C, Lammas DA, Picard C, Dorman SE, Sanal O, et al. Interleukin (IL)-12 and IL-23 are key cytokines for immunity against Salmonella in humans. J Infect Dis. (2004). Nov 15;, 190(10), 1755-7.

[108] Rudner, X. L, Happel, K. I, Young, E. A, Shellito, J. E, & Interleukin-23, I. L. IL-17 cytokine axis in murine Pneumocystis carinii infection. Infect Immun. (2007). Jun;, 75(6), 3055-61.

[109] Shear, N. H, Prinz, J, Papp, K. Langley, R. G, & Gulliver, W. P. Targeting the interleukin-12/23 cytokine family in the treatment of psoriatic disease. J Cutan Med Surg. (2008). Dec;12 Suppl 1:S, 1-10.

[110] Chackerian, A. A, Chen, S. J, Brodie, S. J, Mattson, J. D, Mcclanahan, T. K, Kastelein, R. A, et al. Neutralization or absence of the interleukin-23 pathway does not compromise immunity to mycobacterial infection. Infect Immun. (2006). Nov;, 74(11), 6092-9.

[111] Dumoutier, L, Louahed, J, & Renauld, J. C. Cloning and characterization of IL-10-related T cell-derived inducible factor (IL-TIF), a novel cytokine structurally related to IL-10 and inducible by IL-9. J Immunol. (2000). Feb 15;, 164(4), 1814-9.

[112] Wolk, K, Kunz, S, Asadullah, K, & Sabat, R. Cutting edge: immune cells as sources and targets of the IL-10 family members? J Immunol. (2002). Jun 1;, 168(11), 5397-402.

[113] Nograles, K. E, Zaba, L. C, Shemer, A, Fuentes-duculan, J, Cardinale, I, Kikuchi, T, et al. IL-22-producing "T22" T cells account for upregulated IL-22 in atopic dermatitis despite reduced IL-17-producing TH17 T cells. J Allergy Clin Immunol. (2009). Jun;e2., 123(6), 1244-52.

[114] Duhen, T, Geiger, R, Jarrossay, D, Lanzavecchia, A, & Sallusto, F. Production of interleukin 22 but not interleukin 17 by a subset of human skin-homing memory T cells. Nat Immunol. (2009). Aug;, 10(8), 857-63.

[115] Wolk, K, Haugen, H. S, Xu, W, Witte, E, Waggie, K, Anderson, M, et al. IL-22 and IL-20 are key mediators of the epidermal alterations in psoriasis while IL-17 and IFN-gamma are not. J Mol Med. (2009). May;, 87(5), 523-36.

[116] Wolk, K, Witte, E, Warszawska, K, Schulze-tanzil, G, Witte, K, Philipp, S, et al. The Th17 cytokine IL-22 induces IL-20 production in keratinocytes: A novel immunological cascade with potential relevance in psoriasis. Eur J Immunol. (2009). Oct 14.

[117] Sabat, R, & Wolk, K. Research in practice: IL-22 and IL-20: significance for epithelial homeostasis and psoriasis pathogenesis. J Dtsch Dermatol Ges. (2011). Jan 21.

[118] Boniface, K, Bernard, F. X, Garcia, M, Gurney, A. L, Lecron, J. C, & Morel, F. IL-22 inhibits epidermal differentiation and induces proinflammatory gene expression and migration of human keratinocytes. J Immunol. (2005). Mar 15;, 174(6), 3695-702.

[119] Wolk, K, Kunz, S, Witte, E, Friedrich, M, Asadullah, K, & Sabat, R. IL-22 increases the innate immunity of tissues. Immunity. (2004). Aug;, 21(2), 241-54.

[120] Kotenko, S. V, Izotova, L. S, Mirochnitchenko, O. V, Esterova, E, Dickensheets, H, Donnelly, R. P, et al. Identification of the functional interleukin-22 (IL-22) receptor complex: the IL-10R2 chain (IL-10Rbeta) is a common chain of both the IL-10 and IL-22 (IL-10-related T cell-derived inducible factor, IL-TIF) receptor complexes. J Biol Chem. (2001). Jan 26;, 276(4), 2725-32.

[121] Savan, R, Mcfarland, A. P, Reynolds, D. A, Feigenbaum, L, Ramakrishnan, K, Karwan, M, et al. A novel role for IL-22R1 as a driver of inflammation. Blood. (2011). Jan 13;, 117(2), 575-84.

[122] Jones, B. C, Logsdon, N. J, & Walter, M. R. Structure of IL-22 bound to its high-affinity IL-22R1 chain. Structure. (2008). Sep 10;, 16(9), 1333-44.

[123] Lejeune, D, Dumoutier, L, Constantinescu, S, Kruijer, W, Schuringa, J. J, Renauld, J. C, & Interleukin-22, I. L. activates the JAK/STAT, ERK, JNK, and MAP kinase pathways in a rat hepatoma cell line. Pathways that are shared with and distinct from IL-10. J Biol Chem. (2002). Sep 13;277(37):33676-82., 38.

[124] Horwitz, D. A, Gray, J. D, & Zheng, S. G. The potential of human regulatory T cells generated ex vivo as a treatment for lupus and other chronic inflammatory diseases. Arthritis Res. (2002). , 4(4), 241-6.

[125] Korn, T, Mitsdoerffer, M, & Kuchroo, V. K. Immunological basis for the development of tissue inflammation and organ-specific autoimmunity in animal models of multiple sclerosis. Results Probl Cell Differ. (2010). , 51, 43-74.

[126] Ramsdell, F, & Fowlkes, B. J. Clonal deletion versus clonal anergy: the role of the thymus in inducing self tolerance. Science. (1990). Jun 15;, 248(4961), 1342-8.

[127] Sakaguchi, S, Toda, M, Asano, M, Itoh, M, Morse, S. S, & Sakaguchi, N. T cell-mediated maintenance of natural self-tolerance: its breakdown as a possible cause of various autoimmune diseases. J Autoimmun. (1996). Apr;, 9(2), 211-20.

[128] Sakaguchi, S, Sakaguchi, N, Shimizu, J, Yamazaki, S, Sakihama, T, Itoh, M, et al. Immunologic tolerance maintained by CD25+ CD4+ regulatory T cells: their common role in controlling autoimmunity, tumor immunity, and transplantation tolerance. Immunol Rev. (2001). Aug;, 182, 18-32.

[129] Gershon, R. K, & Kondo, K. Infectious immunological tolerance. Immunology. (1971). Dec;, 21(6), 903-14.

[130] Dorf, M. E, & Benacerraf, B. Suppressor cells and immunoregulation. Annu Rev Immunol. (1984). , 2, 127-57.

[131] Green, D. R, & Webb, D. R. Saying the'S' word in public. Immunol Today. (1993). Nov;, 14(11), 523-5.

[132] Shevach, E. M, Thornton, A, & Suri-payer, E. T lymphocyte-mediated control of autoimmunity. Novartis Found Symp. (1998). discussion 11-30., 215, 200-11.

[133] Belkaid, Y, Blank, R. B, & Suffia, I. Natural regulatory T cells and parasites: a common quest for host homeostasis. Immunol Rev. (2006). Aug;, 212, 287-300.

[134] Weiner, H. L. da Cunha AP, Quintana F, Wu H. Oral tolerance. Immunol Rev. (2011). May;, 241(1), 241-59.

[135] Shehata, I. H, & Elghandour, T. M. A possible pathogenic role of CD4+CD25+ T-regulatory cells in psoriasis. Egypt J Immunol. (2007). , 14(1), 21-31.

[136] Sabat, R, Philipp, S, Hoflich, C, Kreutzer, S, Wallace, E, Asadullah, K, et al. Immunopathogenesis of psoriasis. Exp Dermatol. (2007). Oct;, 16(10), 779-98.

[137] Sugiyama, H, Gyulai, R, Toichi, E, Garaczi, E, Shimada, S, Stevens, S. R, et al. Dysfunctional blood and target tissue CD4+CD25high regulatory T cells in psoriasis: mechanism underlying unrestrained pathogenic effector T cell proliferation. J Immunol. (2005). Jan 1;, 174(1), 164-73.

[138] Wilhelm, A. J, Zabalawi, M, Owen, J. S, Shah, D, Grayson, J. M, Major, A. S, et al. Apolipoprotein A-I modulates regulatory T cells in autoimmune LDLr-/-, ApoA-I-/- mice. J Biol Chem. (2010). Nov 12;, 285(46), 36158-69.

[139] Ortega, C, Fernandez, A. S, Carrillo, J. M, Romero, P, Molina, I. J, Moreno, J. C, et al. IL-17-producing CD8+ T lymphocytes from psoriasis skin plaques are cytotoxic effector cells that secrete Th17-related cytokines. J Leukoc Biol. (2009). Aug;, 86(2), 435-43.

[140] Yu, P, Lee, Y, Liu, W, Krausz, T, Chong, A, Schreiber, H, et al. Intratumor depletion of CD4+ cells unmasks tumor immunogenicity leading to the rejection of late-stage tumors. J Exp Med. (2005). Mar 7;, 201(5), 779-91.

[141] Abrams, J. R, Kelley, S. L, Hayes, E, Kikuchi, T, Brown, M. J, Kang, S, et al. Blockade of T lymphocyte costimulation with cytotoxic T lymphocyte-associated antigen 4-immunoglobulin (CTLA4Ig) reverses the cellular pathology of psoriatic plaques, including the activation of keratinocytes, dendritic cells, and endothelial cells. J Exp Med. (2000). Sep 4;, 192(5), 681-94.

[142] Sewgobind, V. D, Van Der Laan, L. J, Kho, M. M, Kraaijeveld, R, Korevaar, S. S, Mol, W, et al. The calcineurin inhibitor tacrolimus allows the induction of functional CD4CD25 regulatory T cells by rabbit anti-thymocyte globulins. Clin Exp Immunol. (2010). Aug;, 161(2), 364-77.

[143] Vukmanovic-stejic, M, Mcquaid, A, Birch, K. E, Reed, J. R, Macgregor, C, Rustin, M. H, et al. Relative impact of CD4+CD25+ regulatory T cells and tacrolimus on inhibition of T-cell proliferation in patients with atopic dermatitis. Br J Dermatol. (2005). Oct;, 153(4), 750-7.

[144] De Rezende, L. C, Silva, I. V, Rangel, L. B, & Guimaraes, M. C. Regulatory T cell as a target for cancer therapy. Arch Immunol Ther Exp (Warsz). (2010). Jun;, 58(3), 179-90.

[145] Lutsiak, M. E, Semnani, R. T, De Pascalis, R, Kashmiri, S. V, Schlom, J, & Sabzevari, H. Inhibition of CD4(+)25+ T regulatory cell function implicated in enhanced immune response by low-dose cyclophosphamide. Blood. (2005). Apr 1;, 105(7), 2862-8.

[146] Cerullo, V, Diaconu, I, Kangasniemi, L, Rajecki, M, Escutenaire, S, Koski, A, et al. Immunological Effects of Low-dose Cyclophosphamide in Cancer Patients Treated With Oncolytic Adenovirus. Mol Ther. (2011). Jun 14.

[147] Ikezawa, Y, Nakazawa, M, Tamura, C, Takahashi, K, Minami, M, & Ikezawa, Z. Cyclophosphamide decreases the number, percentage and the function of CD25+ CD4+ regulatory T cells, which suppress induction of contact hypersensitivity. J Dermatol Sci. (2005). Aug;, 39(2), 105-12.

[148] Stock, P, Akbari, O, Dekruyff, R. H, & Umetsu, D. T. Respiratory tolerance is inhibited by the administration of corticosteroids. J Immunol. (2005). Dec 1;, 175(11), 7380-7.

[149] Papp, K. A, Leonardi, C, Menter, A, Ortonne, J. P, Krueger, J. G, Kricorian, G, et al. Brodalumab, an anti-interleukin-17-receptor antibody for psoriasis. N Engl J Med. (2012). Mar 29;, 366(13), 1181-9.

[150] Leonardi, C, Matheson, R, Zachariae, C, Cameron, G, Li, L, Edson-heredia, E, et al. Anti-interleukin-17 monoclonal antibody ixekizumab in chronic plaque psoriasis. N Engl J Med. (2012). Mar 29;, 366(13), 1190-9.

[151] Sivamani, R. K, Goodarzi, H, Garcia, M. S, Raychaudhuri, S. P, Wehrli, L. N, Ono, Y, et al. Biologic Therapies in the Treatment of Psoriasis: A Comprehensive Evidence-

Based Basic Science and Clinical Review and a Practical Guide to Tuberculosis Monitoring. Clin Rev Allergy Immunol. (2012). Feb 5.

[152] Kopf, M, Bachmann, M. F, & Marsland, B. J. Averting inflammation by targeting the cytokine environment. Nat Rev Drug Discov. (2010). Sep;, 9(9), 703-18.

Chapter 4

Pathophysiology of Psoriasis: Current Concepts

Hani A. Al-Shobaili and Muhammad Ghaus Qureshi

Additional information is available at the end of the chapter

http://dx.doi.org/10.5772/54113

1. Introduction

The word 'psoriasis', is derived from the Greek word "psora" meaning "itch" or "scurf" or "rash", although most patients suffering from the condition do not complain of itching. It has been known since ancient times and was originally considered a type of leprosy. For quite some time now, it is one of the most common human skin diseases. Up to a few decades back, psoriasis was considered to be a chronic inflammatory dermatosis with albeit, genetic factors involved in the pathogenesis.

It is now considered a multifactorial disorder that has several factors like genetic predisposition, environmental, immunologically mediated inflammation and several modifying factors including obesity, trauma, infection and a possible deficiency of the active forms of vitamin D3. Different subsets of T lymphocytes, antigen presenting cells (APC's), keratinocytes, Langerhans' cells, macrophages, natural killer cells, an array of Th1 type cytokines, certain growth factors like vascular endothelial growth factor (VEGF), keratinocyte growth factor (KGF) etc are involved [1].

Psoriasis was long-considered either a disorder of keratinocyte growth or a chronic inflammation. However, advancement in immunologic techniques and in genetic analyses over the past four decades have resulted in a reappraisal of the pathophysiology involved. Some consider psoriasis as an organ-specific autoimmune disease that is triggered by an activated cellular immune system and is similar to other immune-mediated diseases such as Crohn's disease, rheumatoid arthritis, multiple sclerosis and juvenile-onset diabetes. All of these fit the definition of an autoimmune disease as "a clinical syndrome caused by the activation of T cells and B cells, or both, in the absence of an ongoing infection or other discernable cause" [2]. From the many factors postulated to be involved in the pathophysiology of psoriasis and psoriatic arthritis, it is obvious that the mechanism leading to the development of the symmetrically present discoid plaques with silvery scales, is still not understood clearly. In spite of the plethora of research studies into its pathogenesis, psoriasis still poses a challenge to the scientific community to, once and for all, establish how and why it occurs and consequently to develop the magic drug to treat it.

2. Role of genetic factors

The idea that psoriasis has a genetic component has been there for over a 100 years but it was Lomholt's classic epidemiologic study in 1963 that really established the genetic component in psoriasis. He investigated more than 11,000 of the 30,000 inhabitants of the Faroe islands and studied psoriatic patients and their unaffected relatives. He found a clear genetic basis as the incidence of psoriasis was much greater amongst first- and second degree relatives of patients with psoriasis. Lomholt however, was unable to establish a particular inheritance pattern [3].

Further studies performed in Sweden and later in Germany supported Lomholt's data. Hellgren published extensive data showing the prevalence of psoriasis to be 7.8% in first degree relatives compared with a prevalence of 3.14% in matched controls, and 1.97% in the overall population [4].

3. Racial & geographic variations

Although, psoriasis occurs worldwide, its prevalence is highest in Scandinavian countries and Northern Europe (3%); in contrast, its prevalence in North America and the UK its prevalence is ~2%, while in Japan its prevalence is ~0.2% of the population. Far more interesting is the fact that it is rare in Native American Indians although it is much more prevalent n the USA where 3 million office visits for psoriasis are made each year, costing over $3 billion [5]. It contributes to approximately 1-5% of all skin disorders in Saudi Arabia [6].

3.1. Establishing a genetic component

Over the past two decades or so, cumulative evidence establishing a substantive role for genetic factors in respect to disease susceptibility and expression is based on family based investigations; population based epidemiological studies, association studies with human leucocyte antigens (HLAs), genome-wide linkage scans, and candidate gene studies within and outside the major histocompatibility complex (MHC) region [7 & 8].

3.2. Concordance

There is marked variation in concordance for monozygotic twins in various studies: 35-73% and the concordance never approaching 100% raises the possibility that genetic factor probably act with environmental ones = 12-14 Fitz. The concordance of psoriasis in monozygotic twins approached 65–72%, versus 15–30% in dizygotic twins. Determination of concordance in older twin pairs from a national twin registry in Denmark revealed nearly 90–100% heritability [5]. However, in an Australian study the monozygotic twin concordance rate was found to be considerably lower (35% for monozygotic twins and 12% for dizygotic twins), giving an estimated heritability of 80% [9].

3.3. Inheritance pattern

Despite all the work on psoriasis, the inheritance pattern has not been ascertained and psoriasis has by various authors, been considered a single gene disorder with an autosomal dominant inheritance with its variable expressivity and reduced penetrance or an autosomal recessive disorder because of multiple affected individuals in a family. Patients with more dominance of genetic factors have more severe disease and in a younger age group. The risk for a person of developing psoriasis is 41% if both parents affected; 14% if 1 parent is affected, 6% if one sibling is affected and only 2% when no parent or sibling is affected [10].

However, Swanbeck et al presented empirical data that may be of more relevance for genetic counseling. After assessing over 3000 families in which one or both parents had psoriasis, the calculated lifetime risk of getting psoriasis if no parent, one parent, or both parents have psoriasis was found to be 0.04, 0.28, and 0.65, respectively. If there was already one affected child in the family, the corresponding risks were 0.24, 0.51, and 0.83, respectively [11]. Possession of certain HLA class I antigens, particularly HLA-Cw6, is associated with an earlier age of onset and with a positive family history. This finding led to the proposal that two different forms of psoriasis exist: type I psoriasis, with age of onset before 40 years and HLA-associated, and type II, with age of onset after 40 years and lacking HLA associations, although many patients do not fit into this classification. There is no evidence that type I and type II psoriasis respond differently to different therapies. So far, between 10 and 20 chromosome regions have been proposed to harbour psoriasis genes but less than a handful of genes have been identified. This is due, in part, to their low-risk effects and the limitations in the number of patients and families that have been studied. One locus consistently identified in studies of psoriasis is the class I region of the major histocompatibility locus antigen cluster. However, it's low penetrance — about 10% — indicates that other genetic and environmental factors are also involved. The identity of psoriasis susceptibility 1 (*PSORS1*) remains controversial. Although its association with human leukocyte antigen (HLA) Cw6 and psoriasis was reported more than 25 years age, the extensive linkage disequilibrium across the class I region and its complex evolutionary history has made identification of the susceptibility variant(s) very difficult. Genes within this region lying about 160 kilobases telomeric to HLA-C, such as corneodesmosin (*CDSN*) and the α-helical coiled-coil rod (*HCR*), have been proposed as contenders. A consensus is now beginning to emerge that supports the location of *PSORS1* as being closer to the region harboring HLA-C/HLA-B and excluding *CDSN* and *HCR*. However, whether *PSORS1* is a classical MHC allele, or a regulatory variant within this region, has not yet been agreed upon. Other predisposing polygenes might affect the immune system or be involved in keratinocyte differentiation. Common variants in the SLC9A3R1/NAT9 region and loss of a potential RUNX binding site have been described that could potentially affect regulation of the immune synapse [12].PSORS1 is located in the major histocompatibility complex (MHC, chromosome 6p21.3), home of the

HLA) genes.[17] Multiple HLA alleles have been associated with psoriasis, particularly HLA-B13, HLA-B37, HLA-B46, HLA-B57, HLA-Cw1, HLA-Cw6, HLA-DR7, and HLA-DQ9.[10] Many of these alleles are in linkage disequilibrium with HLA-Cw6 (i.e., found together on the same chromosome more often than would be predicted by chance). HLA-Cw6 has consistently demonstrated the highest relative risk for psoriasis in Caucasian populations [13].

4. Immunological factors in psoriasis

Both innate and acquired immune changes are thought to be responsible for the development of psoriatic plaques. Different types of helper T subsets, dendritic cells, plasmacytoid dendritic cells as well as Langerhans cells have been found to play a role in psoriasis. Research had already suggested the role of T cells in psoriasis. Further studies led to the successful use of T-cell immunosuppressant cyclosporin A in the treatment of psoriasis The concept that T cell activation is a key event in psoriasis was further strengthened with the successful use of anti-T cell specific drugs in the form of anti-CD3 and -CD4 monoclonal antibodies in treatment. There is also the possibility that psoriasis may be an organ-specific autoimmune disease with similarities to rheumatoid arthritis and multiple sclerosis and the recent use of so-called "etio-pathogenetic" drugs like methotrexate, and alefacept suggests autoimmunity as a major factor in pathogenesis. [14].

5. Histologic features of psoriasis and their Immunological basis

Light Microscopic features of psoriasis include three predominant groups of changes: i) epidermal hyperplasia ii) inflammatory infiltrate and iii) vascular changes. All of these changes must be explained satisfactorily by any hypothesis, to withstand a critical scrutiny. The epidermal changes include keratinocyte hyperplasia, an attenuated or absent granular cell layer and impaired keratinocyte differentiation and maturation. The combination of these epidermal changes leads to the thick scaly plaques characteristic of psoriasis [15]. The inflammatory infiltrate in the dermis is seen to invade the epidermis (exocytosis) and is mainly composed of Th1 helper T cells as well as the cytotoxic CD8+ cells. In addition there is an infiltration of neutrophils that go on to form the diagnostic histologic features spongiform pustule of Kogoj and Munro microabscess. The third change is vascular and consists of increased number of the vessels in the superficial vascular plexus with tortuosity of vessels and most interestingly venulization of the capillary network so that the vessels become HEV (High Endothelial Venules) [16].

The presence of T cells in the inflammatory infiltrate in psoriatic plaques obviously indicated an immune-mediated or an autoimmune basis for the pathogenesis of psoriasis. The evidence of an immune basis comes from research in the laboratory with experimental animals as well as from clinical research and particularly the significant regression of the disease with the use immunosuppressive agents like cyclosporine which act against T cells.

http://dx.doi.org/10.5772/54113

6. Mouse models of psoriasis and the immune basis of the disease

There is no animal model where psoriatic lesions may be produced de novo. Initially humanized mouse models in which psoriatic skin was xenografted onto immunodeficient mice was used as a means to study the immune pathways leading to the development and resolution of psoriatic lesions. When non-lesional (normal-looking) skin from psoriatic patients was injected with superantigen-activated leukocytes and subsequently grafted onto these mice, there was development of new lesions on the transplanted skin. This provided strong evidence that T cells play a key role in the pathology of the disease. Later, a new model of xenotransplantation was developed. This entailed non-lesional skin from psoriatic patients being engrafted onto AGR129 mice (lacking T and B cells and with severely impaired NK cell responses). It was seen that the non-lesional skin grafts transplanted onto AGR129 mice spontaneously converted to lesional skin, suggesting that all of the elements required for the development of psoriasis lesions are present in non-lesional skin. This conversion was associated with enhanced proliferation of T cells that are resident in non-lesional skin and increased TNF-α production. All this argued in favor of a dominant role of cytokines and T cells in the pathogenesis indicating an immune or autoimmune basis [17].

Valdmarson et al discovered that an early event in the evolving lesions of guttate psoriasis was an intrepidermal influx of activated T cells that were HLA- DR+, CD4+, while on the other hand, resolving plaques of psoriasis showed a reduced intraepidermal infiltration [18].

However, evidence was produced by other researchers showing that CD8+ T cells were predominant in psoriatic epidermis and that the decrease in the number of these cells was more closely related to resolution of the plaques following treatment. But regardless of the phenotype of these T cells, it was agreed that they were activated and that they were HLA- DR+, expressed the IL-2 receptor CD25 and also secreted cytokines IL-2 and γ-IFN both of which are involved in the activation of T cells [19]. It was also deduced from the presence of activated and proliferating dermal dendritic antigen-presenting cells the presence of activated and proliferating memory T cells, that the signals for these changes were derived from the skin itself [20].

It was also noted by different researchers that the T cells in present in psoriatic plaques of different patterns of psoriasis based on two different groups of cytokines secreted. Mossman for example found that a Th1 profile is indicated by a predominance of IL-2, IL-12 and γ-interferon while a Th2 profile is indicated by the predominance of IL-4, IL-5 and IL-10 [21].

7. Innate immunity in psoriasis

The role of the innate immune system in psoriasis is increasingly seen as important. Neutrophils are found in the stratum corneum of psoriatic skin [22]. Since neutrophils have a short life span (about 3 days), their persistent presence in the epidermis suggests that they are continually recruited. Dendritic cells (DCs) are increased in psoriatic lesions and also appear to play their part in the T-cell response [23 & 24].

Subsets of DCs not usually found in the skin are also observed to be present in psoriatic skin lesions. Plasmacytoid DCs are potent producers of IFN-α, which is thought to be a key cytokine in triggering lesion development, and myeloid DCs, with the ability to secrete TNF-α and inducible nitric oxide synthase, have been also been observed in psoriatic skin. There are increased numbers of mature and activated DCs in psoriatic lesions implying that these cells may be stimulating other aspects of the immune response. Innate immunity is associated with the production of proinflammatory or primary cytokines. The most important of them are IL-1α and TNF-α. The role of IL-1α is unclear as detection in psoriasis lesions has given conflicting results. TNF-α is increased in lesional skin of psoriasis patients and in synovium of patients with psoriatic arthritis [25].

8. Natural Killer (NK) cells and psoriasis

NK cells are lymphocytes that are generally considered to be part of the innate immune system. They are best known for their ability to kill virally infected and cancer cells; however, they also produce a range of cytokines including IFN-γ, TNF-α, and TGF-β. They can be defined phenotypically by the presence of particular surface antigens: either NKp46 or $CD56^{+}CD3^{-}$cells. While the role of NK cells in psoriasis still remains relatively unstudied, there is mounting evidence that these cells may contribute to disease. Ottaviani et al. found that the inflammatory infiltrate into psoriatic skin consisted of 5–8% cells that expressed the NK cell phenotype of $CD56^{+}CD3^{-}$. Most of these were of the $CD56^{bright}$ subset of NK cells. Thought to represent more immature cells, $CD56^{bright}$ cells are less cytotoxic and more proficient at cytokine secretion compared to $CD56^{dim}$ NK cells. The cells present in the infiltrate found by Ottaviani et al. also expressed the activation antigen, CD69, and produced large quantities of IFN-γ *in vitro* in response to IL-2 stimulation. Supernatants from these IL2-stimulated NK cells induced activation of keratinocytes causing upregulation of MHC class I molecules and induction of the expression of ICAM1 and HLA-DR receptors. The keratinocytes were also observed to secrete chemokines that are known to attract NK cells (CXCL10, CCL5, and CCL20) thereby providing a mechanism of NK cell recruitment to the skin [26].

More weight is added to the possibility of a dysregulated immune system playing a role in psoriasis by the impressively good response following treatment with TNF-α neutralizing modalities. For example, one course of infliximab (Remicade®) results in an impressive Psoriasis Activity and Severity Index (PASI) 75 of 80%, meaning that at least 80% of patients have a decrease of at least 75% of their psoriasis skin symptoms [27]

9. Neutrophils and psoriasis

Although psoriasis is a chronic disease, the skin lesions often contain groups of neutrophils within small spongiotic foci in the superficial part of the stratum spinosum of the epidermis as well as intermittently within the stratum corneum. Thus, there is an element of acute inflammation changes in the disease which often persists for decades. Thought to be recruited and subsequently activated by a high gradient of chemotactic factors like chemokines, IL-8 and Gro-a released by the stimulated keratinocytes, and particularly C5a/C5a des-arg produced via the alternative complement pathway. Initially, the presence of neutrophils in psoriatic epidermis was considered a secondary and rather passive phenomenon. However, Terui et al proposed "a neutrophil-associated inflammation-boosting loop" and suggested that this may well explain the localized "acute" inflammatory changes scattered over the "chronic" psoriatic plaques as well as in the acutely inflamed lesions of pustular psoriasis. They proposed that these neutrophils may actively increase the activation of T cells and that the activated T cells in turn release cytokines to stimulate epidermal keratinocytes to produce IL-8 and C3 that facilitates complement activation as well as PMN accumulation. The neutrophils forming the intra-corneal Munro microabscess may also influence keratinocytes to induce disturbances of epidermal keratinization and underlying hyperproliferation. They also express HLA-DR under the influence of IFN-g and GM-CSF in turn to potentiate T cells. Thus, PMNs infiltrating into the lesional skin may play a pivotal role in eliciting the acute inflammatory and hyperplastic responses in classic psoriatic plaques [28].

10. Acquired immunity & psoriasis

In contrast to neutrophils which are not persistently present in all psoriatic lesions, increased numbers of T lymphocytes are a highly consistent finding in psoriasis biopsies. With immunohistochemical staining, T lymphocytes are found interspersed between keratinocytes throughout the epidermis and in somewhat larger quantities in the dermis. In fact, a significant fraction of dermal "mononuclear" inflammatory cells seen in routine sections is due to T cell infiltration. T cell subsets are not uniformly distributed in psoriasis lesions. Epidermal T cells are chiefly CD8+ T cells, with a significant fraction of these cells specialized for homing to epithelia through expression of the integrin aeb7, which binds E-cadherin associated with desmosomes. Dermal T lymphocytes are a mixture of CD4+ and CD8+ cells, with a CD4+ predominance similar to that seen in peripheral blood. Most T cells in skin lesions are memory cells that express cutaneous lymphocyte antigen (CLA), the skin addressin. [27] In contrast, only, 10% of circulating T lymphocytes are CLA+. Hence, CLA+ T cells are impressively and selectively targeted to inflammatory psoriasis lesions [29].

Although a case report in 1979 suggested that cyclosporin A could clear psoriasis, this disease was generally considered to be a primary disorder of keratinocytes in the early eighties. A direct role of T cells in the pathogenesis of psoriasis was first suggested in 1983, and it was independently demonstrated that the eruption of psoriatic skin lesions coincided with epidermal influx of dendritic cells (DCs) and T cells and that resolution of psoriatic lesions during phototherapy was preceded by depletion of T cells, especially from the epidermis. The efficacy of cyclosporin A in psoriasis was subsequently confirmed in two independent studies and trials with anti-CD4 monoclonal antibodies and an interleukin-2-toxin conjugate further supported that psoriasis is a T cell-mediated disease. These T cell-specific treatments resulted in the normalization of the keratinocyte proliferation and epidermal thickening.

The key role of T cells in psoriasis was conclusively demonstrated in 1996 when psoriatic lesions were induced by injecting autologous T cells into uninvolved psoriatic skin transplanted to SCID mice. It was further shown in this model that psoriatic lesions could be induced by injecting purified CD4+ T cells into uninvolved psoriatic skin but no changes were seen when purified CD8+ T cells were injected. Although CD4+ T cells therefore seem to be essential for initiating psoriatic lesions, CD8+ T cells may also have an important role in the pathogenic process as uninvolved psoriatic epidermis contains an increased number of CD8+ T cells that may be able to proliferate locally with the help of IL-7 and IL-15, cytokines that are produced by keratinocytes [30].

11. Pathogenesis of vascular changes in psoriasis

Vascular endothelial growth factor (VEGF) has been implicated in the pathologic angiogenesis observed in psoriasis and other chronic inflammatory skin diseases that are characterized by enhanced expression of VEGF by epidermal keratinocytes and of VEGF receptors by tortuous microvessels in the upper dermis. In addition, the number of mast cells in the upper dermis was significantly increased in transgenic skin. Highly increased leukocyte rolling and adhesion in postcapillary skin venules that were both inhibited after injection of blocking antibodies against E- and P-selectin were also seen in experimental studies. It was also revealed that VEGF is a growth factor specific for blood vessels, but not lymphatic vessels, and that chronic orthotopic overexpression of VEGF in the epidermis is sufficient to induce cardinal features of chronic skin inflammation, providing a molecular link between angiogenesis, mast cell accumulation, and leukocyte recruitment to sites of inflammation.

As early as in the 70s Braverman had done an electron microscopic study of ultrastructure of the capillary loops in the dermal papillae of psoriatic lesions. Normal dermal papillary vessels are arterial in nature but in psoriasis these vessels change to have a venous capillary structure. Following 3 weeks of Goeckerman therapy, the morphology of psoriatic capillary loops changed from venous capillaries to arterial capillaries which are found in the papillae of normal skin. This transformation was observed to begin 48 to 72 hr after the initiation of therapy [31].

Four-fold increase of endothelial microvascular bed is reported in the psoriatic skin but not in normal skin, thus signifying the importance of angiogenesis in psoriasis. Dermal microvascular expansion with abnormal orientation and dilatation of capillaries in the biopsies of the psoriatic skin revealed that the disease was angiogenesis dependent. The keratinocytes in the psoriatic skin lesions were recognized as a source of pro-angiogenic cytokines which induce angiogenesis, namely the vascular endothelial growth factor (VEGF). Other commonly recognized cytokines were endothelial cell stimulating angiogenesis factor (ESAF), tumor necrosis factor-α (TNF-α) and platelet derived growth factors (PDGF) and newly discovered VEGF-C, NGF and vWFr [32].

http://dx.doi.org/10.5772/54113

Psoriatic skin is also characterized by microvascular hyperpermeability and angioproliferation. The hyperplastic epidermis of psoriatic skin expresses strikingly increased amounts of vascular permeability factor (VPF; vascular endothelial growth factor), a selective endothelial cell mitogen that enhances microvascular permeability. Moreover, two VPF receptors, kdr and flt-1, are overexpressed by papillary dermal microvascular endothelial cells. Transforming growth factor alpha (TGF-alpha), a cytokine that is also overexpressed in psoriatic epidermis, induced VPF gene expression by cultured epidermal keratinocytes. VPF secreted by TGF-alpha-stimulated keratinocytes was bioactive, as demonstrated by its mitogenic effect on dermal microvascular endothelial cells in vitro. Together, these findings suggest that TGF-alpha regulates VPF expression in psoriasis by an autocrine mechanism, leading to vascular hyperpermeability and angiogenesis [33].

12. Role of keratinocytes in the pathogenesis of psoriasis

As mentioned earlier, it is the epidermal hyperplasia along with abnormal maturation of keratinocytes that leads to the development of the thick scaly plaques that are so characteristic of psoriasis. Gottlieb AB suggested that the epidermal changes and the inflammatory infiltrate composed of T cells with interspersed neutrophils may be linked together by the cytokines produced by both keratinocytes and leukocytes. Her proposal was based partly, on the fact that epidermal acanthosis and keratinocyte mitoses were often seen in delayed-type hypersensitivity reactions and after the intradermal injection of gamma interferon. Gamma interferon and its induced proteins have been demonstrated in active psoriatic plaques. Increased levels of the keratinocyte autocrine cytokines, transforming growth factor (TGF)-alpha and interleukin (IL)-6, have been detected in active plaques. The apparent overexpression of IL-6 in hyperplastic psoriatic tissue may explain features of psoriasis that link keratinocyte proliferation with immune activation and tissue inflammation. Both IL-6 and gamma interferon increased TGF-alpha expression in normal cultured keratinocytes. Cytokines produced during immune activation and other inflammatory processes may lead to epidermal hyperplasia. This indicated that keratinocytes have an important role to play in the pathogenesis of the disease [34].

The French worker Julien D also suggested most recently that since psoriasis is a polymorphous disease and is an example of an interaction of susceptibility genes, immunological mechanisms and modifying factors, it is unwise to look at the disease as either as an exclusive disorder of the immune system or in an isolated primitive change of the epithelial or stromal skin cells. According to the author, it is more likely that various combinations of selective abnormalities of these two compartments give rise to the psoriatic phenotype. Indeed, if in one hand T-cells are essential in the development of psoriatic plaques, the role of innate immunity in this process is better recognized, and numerous psoriasis susceptibility genes are linked to immunity, on the other hand some susceptibility factors related to primitive abnormalities of keratinocytes and some of the most recent murine models of psoriasis are based on modifications targeted to the keratinocytes [35].

In an exploration into the biochemical basis of the psoriatic pathway, Grove T, found anomalies in protein expression as the basis for abnormal differentiation and hyperproliferation of the keratinocytes in psoriatic lesions. At least six markers of abnormal keratinocyte differentiation have been found, and all have implications in the pathogenesis of the disease. These include aberrations of keratinocyte transglutaminase type I (TGase K), skin-derived antileukoproteinase (SKALP), migration inhibitory factor-related protein-8 (MRP-8), Involucrin, Filaggrin and keratin expression. Several possible biochemical causes for the overproduction of the keratinocytes have been found in psoriatic skin: epidermal growth factor (EGF), bone morphogenetic protein-6 (BMP-6), transforming growth factor-alpha (TGF-a), ornithine decarboxylase, activating protein (AP1) and mitogen-activated protein kinase (MAPK) [36].

13. Cytokines and chemokines in the pathogenesis of psoriasis

Once T cells are activated following possible encounters with unknown antigen, they release cytokines specific for T-helper type 1 (TH1) cells. These cells in turn, play a key role in the pathogenesis of psoriasis. Both activated CD4+ and CD8+ T lymphocytes produce TH1 cytokines. Key TH1-type cytokines involved in the pathogenesis of psoriasis are IFN-y, interleukin (IL)-2, and TNF-a. IL-2 stimulates T-lymphocyte growth, and IL-2 treatment is associated with psoriasis flares. IFN-y may inhibit apoptosis of keratinocytes by stimulating expression of the anti-apoptotic protein Bcl-x in these cells. This may be the key to the keratinocyte hyperplasia in psoriatic lesions along with TNF-α. The latter is also thought to be responsible for setting forth the release of proinflammatory cytokines from T lymphocytes and macrophages, of chemokines from macrophages, and of adhesion molecules from vascular endothelial cells. In addition, TH1 cytokines cause the release of cytokines from other cells [37]. Although the evidence for the Th1 profile was strong, IFN-γ, TNF-α, and IL-12, but not IL-4, IL-5, or IL-10, were also demonstrated within psoriatic lesions at the mRNA and protein levels. This suggested synergy between IFN-γ and TNF-α with regard to production of adhesion molecules such as ICAM-1, and chemotactic polypeptides such as IL-8 or monocyte chemotactic activating factor-1 (MCAF-1) [38]. Chemokines and chemokine receptors were also discovered to be involved in the immunopathogenesis of psoriasis. These include among many others, CCL17, MIG, CXCL9 and RANTES (CCL5). In addition, nitric oxide is present, which may contribute to an angiogenic tissue reaction, accompanied by many growth factors present at elevated levels within psoriatic plaques, including TGF-α, IGF-1, keratinocyte growth factor (KGF), VEGF, nerve growth factor (NGF), amphiregulin, and IL-20 [39].

14. Environmental factors and psoriasis

With evidence of a genetic background but the with the confounding lack of 100% concordance in monozygotic twin studies and with the eruptions of guttate psoriasis often being preceded by a streptococcus pyogenes infection as well as the wealth of studies pointing to immune-mediated (possibly autoimmune-mediated) inflammation, it is no wonder that a complex disease like psoriasis has known to be associated with or possibly precipitated by environmental factors. These environmental trigger factors can be mechanical injury, ultraviolet, and chemical injury; various infections; prescription drug use; psychological stress; smoking; and other factors. The most compelling of these is infection with group A streptococci. Streptococcal throat infections frequently precede outbreaks of guttate psoriasis which can then lead to chronic plaque psoriasis. Furthermore, guttate psoriasis is more common in individuals with a family history of plaque psoriasis. A recent study of 29 patients from the UK revealed that all patients with guttate psoriasis carried the HLA-Cw*0602 allele.These same HLA associations are seen in chronic plaque psoriasis, which may also be aggravated by infection. Patients with psoriasis may also have different clinical features depending on whether they are HLA-Cw6 positive or negative. Besides possibly having a lower age of onset, HLA-Cw*0602 positive patients are reported to have more extensive plaques on their arms, legs, and trunk, more severe disease, higher incidence of the Koebner phenomenon, reported more often that their psoriasis got worse during or after throat infections, and more often had a favorable response to sunlight. In contrast, dystrophic nail changes and psoriatic arthritis are reported to be more common in Cw6-negative patients [40].

Deluvio et al (2006) explored the relationship of Streptococcus pyogenes angina with psoriasis. Using TCR analysis, they tried to identify a link between streptococcal angina and the T cell-mediated autoimmune response in psoriasis. They compared the TCR usage of psoriatic skin lesions, blood, tonsils, and tonsillar T cells fractionated according to the expression of the skin address in "cutaneous lymphocyte-associated Ag" (CLA). They found that clones of T cells in the throat of at least one of their three streptococcal patients were similar to the T cell clones in the psoriatic lesion. Because, after tonsillectomy psoriasis cleared in all three of their patients they concluded that T cells may connect psoriatic inflammation to streptococcal angina. They suggest that the chronic streptococcal immune stimulus within the tonsils could act as a source for pathogenic T cells in poststreptococcal disorders, and they may help to explain why eliminating this source with tonsillectomy may improve streptococcal-induced sequelae [41].

15. Koebner phenomenon

The Koebner phenomenon is defined as 'the development of psoriasis at sites of traumatized skin'. The 'all-or-none principle' means that, if psoriasis occurs in one area of injury, all injured areas develop psoriasis or vice versa. This principle was however, disproved by Kalayciyan et al who did a study on sixty-two patients with psoriasis. The medial aspects of both forearms, devoid of lesions, were pricked using two sets of five 30-gauge needles at an angle of 30 degrees, with 2-cm intervals. On days 14 and 28, the patients' forearms were checked for the presence of a typical psoriatic plaque of white scales on an erythematous papule. On day 28, 45 patients (72.5%) had a negative Koebner response in all prick sites whereas 1 patient (1.6%) had psoriatic papules in 10 out of 10 prick sites. The rest of the patients (n = 16, 25.8%) had between 1 and 9 papules in number. This suggests that the 'all or none' principle does not work in psoriatic patients with Koebner phenomenon [42].

16. Conclusion

For decades, the ongoing controversy on the molecular nature, choreography and hierarchy of these complex interactions e.g., between epidermal keratinocytes, T cells, neutrophils, endothelial cells and sensory nerves has served as a driving force propelling investigative dermatology to ever-new horizons. There is no question that advances in understanding the cellular immunology and biology of psoriasis, when coupled with the biotechnology revolution and rapid advances derived from human genetic studies of autoimmunity, have enhanced insights into the cause and treatment of psoriasis.

The disease starts with the activation of T lymphocyte with an unknown antigen or gene product. T cell activation depends on its binding with APC (antigen presenting cell). T cells express the cell receptor known as TCR (T cell receptor), which recognizes the peptide being presented by the APC in the grove of MHC complex. The antigen stimulated activation leads to the conversion of naive T-cells into an antigen specific cell, which may develop into a memory cell that circulate in the body. After the activation of T cells, a cascade of cytokines viz. GMCSF (granulocyte macrophage colony stimulating factor), EGF, IL-1, IL-6, IL-8, IL-12, IL-17, IL-23, Fractalkine, TNF-α etc. are secreted by the activated T Cells. Due to effect of these cytokines there is keratinocyte proliferation, neutrophil migration, potentiation of Th-1 type response, angiogenesis, up-regulation of adhesion molecule and epidermal hyperplasia [43].

Author details

Hani A. Al-Shobaili[1] and Muhammad Ghaus Qureshi[2]

1 Department of Dermatology, College of Medicine, Qassim University, Buraidah, Saudi Arabia

2 Department of Pathology, College of Medicine, Qassim University, Buraidah, Saudi Arabia

References

[1] Das RP, Jain AK, Ramesh V. Current concepts in the pathogenesis of psoriasis. Indian J Dermatol 2009;54:7-12

[2] (Lowes MA, Bowcock AM & Krueger JG. Review Article: Pathogenesis and therapy of psoriasis. Nature 445; 866-73).

[3] Lomholt G. Psoriasis: Prevalence, Spontaneous Course and Genetics. A Census Study on the Prevalence of Skin Diseases on the Faroe Islands. Copenhagen: GEC Gad, 1963: 31–3.

[4] Hellgren L. Psoriasis: The Prevalence in Sex, Age and Occupational Groups in Total Populations in Sweden. Morphology, Inheritance and Association with Other Skin and Rheumatic Diseases. Stockholm: Almqvist & Wiksell, 1967: 19–53.

[5] Christophers, E. and Krueger, G. (eds) (1987) Psoriasis. McGraw-Hill, New York.

[6] Al Shobili HA, Shahzad M, Al-Marshood A, Khalil A, Settin A and Barrimah I. Genetic Background of Psoriasis. Qassim University IJHS Vol. 4 No. 1 (May 2010)

[7] Rahman P, Gladman DD, Schentag C and Petronis A. Excessive paternal transmission in psoriatic arthritis. Arthritis Rheum. 1999;42:1228–31

[8] Al Shobili HA, Shahzad M, Al-Marshood A, Khalil A, Settin A and Barrimah I. Genetic Background of Psoriasis. Qassim University IJHS Vol. 4 No. 1 (May 2010)

[9] Duffy, D.L., Spelman, L.S. and Martin, N.G. (1993) Psoriasis in Australian twins.J. Am. Acad. Dermatol., 29, 428–434.

[10] Andressen C, Henseler T. Inheritance of psoriasis. Analysis of 2035 family histories. Hautarzt 33 (4): 214-217, 1982.

[11] Al Shobili HA, Shahzad M, Al-Marshood A, Khalil A, Settin A and Barrimah I. Genetic Background of Psoriasis. Qassim University IJHS Vol. 4 No. 1 (May 2010)

[12] (Lowes MA, Bowcock AM & Krueger JG. Review Article: Pathogenesis and therapy of psoriasis. Nature 445; 866-73).

[13] Shobili HA, Shahzad M, Al-Marshood A, Khalil A, Settin A and Barrimah I. Genetic Background of Psoriasis. Qassim University IJHS Vol. 4 No. 1 (May 2010)

[14] Bos JD and De Rie MA. The pathogenesis of psoriasis: immunological facts and speculations. Immunology Today, Volume 20, Number 1, 1 January 1999, pp. 40-46(7)

[15] Barker JNWN. The pathophysiology of psoriasis. Lancet 1991, 338;: 227-30).

[16] Griffiths CE and Voorhees JJ. Psoriasis, T cells and autoimmunity, J R Soc Med. 1996; 89(6): 315-319.

[17] Leanne M. Johnson-Huang, Michelle A. Lowes, and James G. Krueger, Putting together the psoriasis puzzle: an update on developing targeted therapies. Dis Model Mech. 2012 July; 5(4): 423–433.

[18] Valdmarson H, Baker BS, Jansdottir I, Fry L. Psoriasis: A disease of abnormal keratinocyte proliferation induced by T lymphocytes. Immunol Today 1986; 7: 256-9).

[19] de Boer OJ, van der Loos CM, Hamerlinck F, Bos JD, Das PK. Reappraisal of in-situ immunophenotypic analysis of psoriatic skin: interaction of activated HLA- DR+ im-

munocompetent cells and endothelial cells is a major feature of psoriatic lesions. Arch of Dermatol Res 1994; 286: 87-96).

[20] Griffiths CE and Voorhees JJ. Psoriasis, T cells and autoimmunity, J R Soc Med. 1996; 89(6): 315-319).

[21] Mossman TR, Cherwinki H, Bond MW, Giedlin MA, Coffman RL., Two types of murine helper T cell clones I. Definition according to profiles of lymphokine activities and secreted proteins. J Immunol 1986; 136: 2348-57.

[22] Lowes MA, Bowcock AM, Krueger JG. Pathogenesis and therapy of psoriasis. Nature. 2007;445(7130):866–873.

[23] Nestle FO, Kaplan DH, Barker J. Mechanisms of disease: psoriasis. The The New England Journal of Medicine. 2009;361(5):444–509.

[24] Lowes MA, Bowcock AM, Krueger JG. Pathogenesis and therapy of psoriasis. Nature. 2007;445(7130):866–873.

[25] Bos, J.D., De Rie, M.A., Teunissen, M.B.M. and Piskin, G. (2005), Psoriasis: dysregulation of innate immunity. British Journal of Dermatology, 152: 1098–1107

[26] Ottaviani C, Nasorri F, Bedini C, de Pità O, Girolomoni G, Cavani A. CD56brightCD16(-) NK cells accumulate in psoriatic skin in response to CXCL10 and CCL5 and exacerbate skin inflammation. European Journal of Immunology. 2006;36(1):118–128

[27] Bos, J.D., De Rie, M.A., Teunissen, M.B.M. and Piskin, G. (2005), Psoriasis: dysregulation of innate immunity. British Journal of Dermatology, 152: 1098–1107

[28] Terui T, Ozawa M, Tagami H. Role of neutrophils in induction of acute inflammation in T-cell-mediated immune dermatosis, psoriasis: A neutrophil-associated inflammation-boosting loop. Exp Dermatol 2000: 9: 1–10

[29] Krueger J G, Bowcock AM. Psoriasis pathophysiology: current concepts of pathogenesis. Ann Rheum Dis 2005;64(Suppl II):ii30–ii36.

[30] Gudjonsson JE, Johnston A, Sigmundsdottir H, and Valdimarsson H. Immunopathogenic mechanisms in psoriasis. Clin Exp Immunol. 2004 January; 135(1): 1–8.

[31] Braverman IM, Yen A. Ultrastructure of the capillary loops in the dermal papillae of psoriasis.. J Invest Dermatol. 1977 Jan;68(1):53-60

[32] Liew SC, Das-Gupta E, Chakravarthi S, Wong SF, Lee N, Safdar N, Jamil A.Differential expression of the angiogenesis growth factors in psoriasis vulgaris. BMC Res Notes. 2012 Jul 3;5:201.

[33] Detmar M, Brown LF, Claffey KP, Yeo KT, Kocher O, Jackman RW, Berse B, Dvorak HF. Overexpression of vascular permeability factor/vascular endothelial growth factor and its receptors in psoriasis. J Exp Med. 1994 Sep 1;180(3):1141-6.

[34] Gottlieb AB.Immunologic mechanisms in psoriasis. J Invest Dermatol. 1990 Nov;95(5 Suppl):18S-19S.

[35] Julien D. Pathogenesis of psoriasis. Ann Dermatol Venereol. 2012 Apr;139 Suppl 2:S68-72

[36] Grove T. The Pathogenesis of Psoriasis: Biochemical Aspects. Biological & Biomedical Sciences. Issue 1, June 2001.

[37] Krueger G and Ellis CN. Psoriasis—recent advances in understanding its pathogenesis and treatment. J Am Acad Dermatol 2005; 53:S94-100

[38] Nickoloff BJ and Nestle FO. Recent insights into the immunopathogenesis of psoriasis provide new therapeutic opportunities. J Clin Invest. 2004 June 15; 113(12): 1664–1675.

[39] Krueger JG. The immunologic basis for the treatment of psoriasis with new biologic agents. J Am Acad Dermatol. 2002 Jan;46(1):1-23.

[40] Bowcock AM and Barker JN. Genetics of psoriasis: the potential impact on new therapies. Journal of the American Academy of Dermatology Volume 49, Issue 2, Supplement, August 2003, Pages 51–56

[41] Diluvio L, Vollmer S, Besgen P, Ellwart JW, Chimenti S, Prinz JC. Identical TCR beta-chain rearrangements in streptococcal angina and skin lesions of patients with psoriasis vulgaris. J Immunol. 2006 Jun 1;176(11):7104-11.

[42] Kalayciyan A, Aydemir EH, Kotogyan A. Experimental Koebner phenomenon in patients with psoriasis. Dermatology. 2007;215(2):114-7.

[43] Das RP, Jain AK, Ramesh V. Current concepts in the pathogenesis of psoriasis. Indian J Dermatol 2009;54:7-12

Chapter 5

Psoriasis: A Disease of Systemic Inflammation with Comorbidities

Sibel Dogan and Nilgün Atakan

Additional information is available at the end of the chapter

http://dx.doi.org/10.5772/54347

1. Introduction

Psoriasis is a chronic disease which affects 1 to 3% of different ethnic populations [1]. As well as the size of the affected population, the social and emotional burden brought by the stigmatization of psoriasis caused serious innovation to the pathogenesis and treatment of the disease.

The majority of the current data about psoriasis is about immune system elements and role of inflammation in the pathogenesis. The development of psoriasis is associated with genetic predisposition which has a basis of T cell activation secondary to dermal inflammation with abnormal keratinocyte proliferation. Tumor necrosis factor alpha (TNF-α), interferon gama (IFN-γ), and interleukin (IL)-8 which are secreted by T lymphocytes, keratinocytes and inflammatory cells polarize type 1 T lymphocytic pathway and lead to the migration of polymorphonuclear leukocytes to the epidermis predominantly [2]. Upregulation of HLADR, intercellular adhesion molecule-1 and E-selectin activates CD2+, CD3+, CD5+, CLA+, CD45RO, HLA-DR, CD25 (IL-2 receptor) and CD27 expressing T cells [2]. Migration and accumulation of inflammatory cells in the epidermis destroyes the basal membrane and desmosomes. In response to the damage, mitogenic cyokines are secreted and a similar process to wound healing results in rapid cell cycling and rapid maturation of keratinocytes [1, 2, 3].The constant inflammatory cell chemotaxis and cytokine release causes the chronic clinical course with recurrent lesions.

Inflammation is described as a complex physiologic defense mechanism consisting of local changes in hemodinamy, increase in microvascular permeability and a series of intracellular reactions [4]. The autoimmune connective diseases are mainly defined as the prototype of inflammatory diseases. Recently, atherosclerosis, obesity and diabetes mellitus are included in inflammatory disease category because they are also proved to cause secondary tissue damage by inflammatory mechanisms [4, 5].

In psoriasis, T cells together with their cytokines and chemokines are shown to induce serious inflammation by Th1- and Th17-driven immune response including IL-20, IL-23, IL-12, IL-17 and IL-22 [2, 3, 4, 5]. Lately psoriasis is assumed as an immune mediated inflammatory disease and psoriatic patients are exposed to the systemic effects of the inflammation [5].

2. Psoriasis as a systemic disease

Psoriatic patients were shown to have inceased levels of circulating Th1-type cytokines, soluble adhesion molecules, vascular endothelial growth factor (VEGF), epidermal growth factor (EGF) and acute phase reactants [2, 3, 4, 5, 6]. As a systemic inflammatory disease, more specific and sensitive markers are thought to be beneficial in monitorizing the systemic inflammation observed in psoriasis where they can be used to predict the development risk of secondary inflammatory diseases; psoriatic comorbidities.

The comorbidities of psoriasis are listed as obesity/metabolic syndrome, autoimmune diseases, psychiatric diseases, cardiovascular diseases, sleep apnea, cancer/lymphoma, non-alcoholic steatohepatitis (NASH) and chronic obstructive pulmonary disease (COPD) [7, 8, 9, 10, 11, 12]. In this chapter, the comorbidities which are especially related with systemic inflammation of psoriasis will be discussed in more detail.

2.1. Psoriasis and systemic inflammatory markers

The studies conducted for the definition of inflammatory process of psoriasis helped to perform the exact measurements for proinflammatory cytokines such as IL-1 and TNF-α, adhesion molecules as intracellular adhesion molecule-1 (ICAM-1) and selectines, IL-6 and hepatic acute phase reactants as C reactive protein (CRP) [13, 14].

CRP testing is particularly important and it is also been proved to be risk predictor for the development of cardiovasculary diseases [15, 16, 17, 18].

2.1.1. C reactive protein

C reactive protein was first defined by Tillett and Francis as a protein developed against carbonhydrate component of streptococcus pneumonia capsule in the serum of patients with pneumonia and named as carbonhydrate reactive protein [19]. CRP is a non-glycolised pentameric protein made by hepatocytes with a molecular weight of 118 kilodaltons (kD). The molecule is known as a major acute phase reactant which increases rapidly after infections or tissue damage, widely used as a laboratory parameter for the follow-up of inflammatory and infectious disease activity and is accepted as a very sensitive inflammatory marker [17, 18, 19]. Blood levels of CRP can increase 100 times in the first 24 hours and can decrease to normal levels soon after treatment or spontaneous healing. Therefore CRP is a valuable laboratory parameter for infections, tissue damage and inflammation. Standard measurements of CRP levels can detect plasma levels of 3-8 mg/l CRP levels and healthy individuals have blood levels of CRP under 2 mg/l. New laboratory methods for the measurement of CRP have been developed and these sensitive CRP measurements can detect lower levels of CRP which are significantly related to certain inflammatory diseases and cardiovascular diseases[16, 17, 18, 19].

The synthesis of CRP is mainly controlled by IL-6 but IL-1 and TNF-α may influence CRP levels as well and increase of CRP in blood and other body fluids is a constant result of these proinlammatory cytokines [15,16]. In this aspect, serum CRP is an indirect marker of proinflammtory cytokine activity. As a fact, CRP plays a role in host's immune defense. It binds to the phosphocoline on the surface of the microorganisms preparing them for phagocytosis and lysis. It also activates complement system by binding to LDL on atherosclerotic plaques and induces inflammation [15, 16]. CRP is also shown to increase the expression of tissue factor on macrophages resuting trombosis. As a classic acute phase marker, CRP induces monocyte-macrophage migration, expression of tissue factor with adhesion molecules and monocyte chemotactic protein-1 [15, 16, 17]. By all of these features, CRP is assumed to increase ischemic myocard damage by participating aterosclerotic pathogenesis.

CRP levels raise as a part of ischemia related acute phase response. Among the plasma markers, CRP is widely used to assess cardiovascular risk. Highly sensitive methods of CRP measurements showed that even levels of CRP within normal ranges may have predictive value in acute coronary syndromes. Sensitive CRP levels are found significantly high when ruptured aterom plaques exist. Recent studies also reveal that there is a strong independent relationship between CRP and future cardiovascular events. American Heart Association and Center for Disease Control (CDC) reported that sensitive CRP is a risk marker for coronary artery diseases [19, 20, 21, 22, 23, 24].

Recent studies showed that psoriatic patients have increased CRP levels and it was also suggested that psoriasis is a systemic inflammatory disease preparing a convenient environment for cardiovascular diseases and comorbidities. The theraupatic modalities of psoriasis are also started to be investigated for their efficacies for lowering CRP levels. Metothrexate (MTX) is found to be efficient in decreasing CRP levels in rheumatoid arthritis (RA) [25, 26]. In fact, MTX therapy reduced the incidence of vascular disease in patients with psoriasis or RA and it was hypothesized that this effect is caused by the drug's anti-inflammatory property [27]. Cyclosporine was efficient as metothraxate and etanercept in decreasing CRP levels in psoriatic arthiritis [26, 28]. In a recent study, patients with higher sensitive CRP levels were found to have a better response to cyclosporine therapy [29]. TNF-α inhibitors managed to decrease CRP levels in patients with psoriasis and RA [30, 31]. However, in a meta-analysis investigating association between biologic therapies and cardiovascular events, there was no significant difference in the rate of major cardiovascular events observed in patients receiving anti-IL-12/IL-23 antibodies or anti-TNF-α treatments compared with placebo [32].

Effective treatment of severe psoriasis is thought to be crucial in avoiding systemic inflammatory response although not determined precisely. Therefore psoriatic therapies must also aim the control of a systemic inflammatory disease which is accepted as a predisposition to cardiovasculary diseases. As well as to obtain healthy skin barier and to increase the severely impaired quality of life, the monitorization and control of systemic inflammation must be aimed. CRP seems to promise an efficient option for this aim.

2.1.2. Other inflammatory markers

In addition to CRP, there are a few investigated serum inflammatory markers in psoriasis. Serum amyloid A (SAA) protein is the precursor of amyloid fibrils which deposit in secondary amyloidosis. It is primerely synthesized as an acute inflammatory reactant from the liver with a molecular weight of 11685 D. Acute inflammatory markers are known to be regulated by hormones, cytokines derived from adipose tissue and synthesized in liver [33, 34]. Adipose tissue is known as the most important source of IL-6 in body and accepted to play a key role in SAA and CRP synthesis. SAA release is likewise increased by IL-1, IL-6 and TNF- α. SAA has a wide level range, it raises rapidly and decreases so soon after infections and enables to represent the acute inflammatory process better than CRP [36]. SAA is a protein which is also a member of high density lipoproteins (HDL) and is synthesized as the predominant apolipoprotein on the plasma HDL particules within the acute inflammatory process. SAA is also produced by synovial fibroblasts and induce colleganase. Immune system cells are attracted by SAA to related sites of inflammation [37].

Inflammatory reactants are released in a coordinated order with systemic and metabolic changes as a response to tissue damage and infection. SAA is a major component of acute inflammatory response. In a similar way to CRP, SAA rises in the serum after infection, inflammation, tissue damage and stress. It is shown to raise in chronic infectious diseases like tuberculosis, lepra, in autoimmune diseases like RA and systemic lupus erythematosus, in kidney transplant rejection, benign monoclonal gammopathy and malign diseases [17, 37].

The increased SAA within acute inflammatory process replaces with apolipoprotein A-1 and decreases the HDL mediated cholesterole entry to the liver cells which is supported by inceased levels of SAA in coronary artery disease patients. High sensitive CRP and SAA are related with vasculary wall inflammation and accepted as predictors of coronary vascular events. In a study in 1999 SAA is found as an independent risk factor for cardiovasculary diseases [37]. In another study SAA was found as a strong predictor for cardiovasculary diseases [22, 37, 38]. In a recent study involving severe psoriatic patients, SAA was found significantly higher in patients with severe psoriasis compared to a sex and age matched control group [39].

Other inflammatory markers recently investigated in psoriasis are platelet-derived microparticles, soluble P-selectin, adiponectins, lectins, haptoglobins, ceruloplasmin, α1- antitrypsin, chitinase 3-like protein 1 (YKL-40, CHI3L1) and serum lipocalin-2 [40, 41, 42, 43].

2.2. Psoriasis and comorbidities

Diseases included as psoriatic comorbidities are obesity/metabolic syndrome, autoimmune diseases, psychiatric diseases cardiovascular diseases, sleep apnea, cancer/lymphoma,

NASH and COPD. In this chapter, the systemic inflammation related comorbidities of psoriasis will be discussed.

2.2.1. *Psoriasis and obesity/metabolic syndrome*

Adipose tissue is known as the most important source of IL-6 in body. Inflammation is mainly controlled by hormones, cytokines derived from adipose tissue and liver by IL-1, IL-6 and TNF- α. Common cytokine pathways are responsible for both psoriasis and obesity but it is yet to be answered which pathology comes first when psoriasis-associated obesity and the metabolic syndrome is considered. It is also not revealed if the diseases are concurrent in a convenient genetic background [44, 45, 46].

Obesity and metabolic syndrome are correlated with increased risk for coronary heart disease. The metabolic syndrome is in fact a group of risk factors which are listed as insulin resistance or glucose intolerance, abdominal/visceral obesity, dyslipidemia (high triglycerides, low HDL-C, high LDL-C), elevated blood pressure, prothrombotic state (high fibrinogen or PAI-1) and proinflammatory state (elevated CRP, TNF- α, IL-6). Several components of metabolic syncrome has been shown to be frequent in psoriatic patients [47]. In a study of 581 moderate-severe psoriasis patients, an increased prevalence was found for metabolic syndrome (OR=5.29), psoriasis patients were more likely to have diabetes mellitus, hypertension, hyperlipidemia, coronary heart disease and they were also more likely to be smokers [48].

Despite the well documentation in adults, there is a few data for obesity/metabolic syndrome in pediatric psoriasis patient population. Augustin et al found a higher prevalence of hyperlipidemia, diabetes, hypertension and obesity in children with psoriasis than the controls retropectively [49]. Koebrick et al showed a significant association between increasing weight and psoriasis in children in a cross-sectional study [50]. In a study by Au et al it was suggested that metabolic syndrome occurs more frequently in pediatric patients with psoriasis [51]. It is assumed that children with psoriasis have excess adiposity and are at risk for associated complications.

2.2.2. *Psoriasis and cardiovascular diseases*

Recent studies show that local and systemic inflammation plays a big role in the pathogenesis of coronary artery diseases (CAD). Bhagat and Vallance has shown that TNF- α and IL- 1 causes a transient reversible endothelium disfunction in humans [13]. High levels of IL- 6 and soluable IL- 2 are shown to be associated with impaired microvasculary functions. A big part of TNF- α induced mechanisms causes endothelium disfunction. TNF- α raises the expression of adhesion molecules. After the exposition of endothelial cells to TNF- α, polimorphonuclear cells migrate to vasculary structures. In fact, TNF- α supports the adhesion and invasion of dendritic cells to vascular walls. After the induction of the dendritic cells, T cells, monocytes and macrophages get activated and produce inflammation by cytokine production. High levels of TNF- α stimulates nitric oxide synthase (NOS) in human endothelium cells. This molecule is known to cause free radical production in neutrophils, smooth muscle cells in the vessels and endothelium. TNF-α induced oxidative stress causes the apopitosis of endothelial cells [13,14]. All of this data shows that endothelial cells are the target of cytokines and other vessel cells. The prolonged exposition of endothelial cells to inflammatory cytokines and oxidative stress results in acceleration of apopitosis, development of trombus and formation of aterosclerotic plaque.

Patients with psoriasis have an increased prevalence of risk factors for CAD. Psoriatic patients who are characterised with elevated TNF- α levels have a significant higher frequency of CAD, pulmonary emboli and cerebrovasculary diseases [52, 53, 54, 55].

Patients with moderate to severe psoriasis have an increased prevalence of CAD and an increased risk for myocardial infarction. In a cohort study by Ahlehoff et al, patients with psoriasis showed a disease severity-dependent increased risk of ischaemic stroke and there was an association between psoriasis and atrial fibrillation [54]. In a cohort study of general practice research database, severe psoriasis was found as a risk factor for major adverse cardiac events (hazard ratio 1.53; 95% confidence interval, 1.26-1.85) after adjusting for age, gender, diabetes, hypertension, tobacco use, and hyperlipidemia. Severe psoriasis added 6.2% absolute risk of major adverse cardiac events.[55] Gelfand et al used the General Practice Research Database (GPRD) to determine if psoriasis is an independent risk factor for myocardial infarction. The study included 3827 (2.9%) severe psoriatic patients with a mean follow-up period of 5.4 years. A significant relationship was shown between the cardiovasculary disease risk and psoriasis duration and severity. An increased incidence of acute myocardial infarction (AMI) in patients with psoriasis was found and the AMI rate was highest in patients with severe psoriasis [56]. Psoriatic patients had a x2.6 increased risk for occlusive vasculary disease and x1.6 increased risk for venous occlusion compared to healthy population Psoriatic patients are also shown to have increased levels of aterotrombotic markers like fibrinogen and plasminogen activator inhibitor-1 (PAI-1) [57].

As well as systemic inflammation, other possible suggested mechanisms for CAD comorbidity of psoriasis are increased prevalence of common CAD risk factors in psoriasis patients and antipsoriatic medications are suspected (cyclosporine, acitretin) for their adverse CAD risk profiles (e.g., elevation of blood pressure, elevation of serum levels of lipids).

3. Conclusion

Psoriasis is associated with multiple CAD risk factors. In fact it is suggested as an independent risk factor for CAD. Obesity and metabolic syndrome are also common in both pediatric and adult psoriatic patients. As a systemic inflammatory disease with important life threatening comorbidities, there is a need for a systematic and complementary understanding of medical care for psoriasis. Screening guidelines for especially severe psoriatic patients has to be reviewed for susceptibility risk factors for the common comorbidities. The approach to psoriasis may also include not only dermatology but also cardiology, rheumatology, and endocrinology assessments at certain points.

Author details

Sibel Dogan[1*] and Nilgün Atakan[2]

*Address all correspondence to: sibel.dogan@hacettepe.edu.tr

1 Bayrampaşa State Hospital, Clinic of Dermatology and Venerology, İstanbul, Turkey

2 Hacettepe University, Faculty of Medicine, Department of Dermatology and Venerology, Ankara, Turkey

References

[1] Gudjonsson JE, Elder JT. Psoriasis. In: Wolff K, Lowell AG, Stephen I (eds). Fitzpatrick's dermatology in general medicine. 7th ed. McGraw-Hill, NewYork. 2008.

[2] Guttman-Yassky E, Krueger J.G. Psoriasis: evolution of pathogenic concepts and new therapies through phases of translational research. British Journal of Dermatology. 2007; 157 1103–1115.

[3] Enno C, Mrowietz U. Psoriasis. In: Braun-Falco O, Plewig G, Wolff HH, Burgdorf WHC (eds). Braun-Falco's Dermatology. 3rd ed. Springer, New York. 2009.

[4] Gaspari AA. Innate and adaptive immunity and the pathophysiology of psoriasis. Journal of the American Academy of Dermatology. 2006;54 67-80.

[5] Prinz JC. The role of T cells in psoriasis. Journal of European Academy of Dermatology Venerology. 2003;17 257-70.

[6] Kaur S, Zimmer K, Leping V, Zilmer M. Comparative study of systemic inflammatory responses in psoriasis vulgaris and mild to moderate allergic contact dermatitis. Dermatology. 2012; 1.-8.

[7] Henseler T, Christophers E. Disease concomitance in psoriasis. Journal of American Academy of Dermatology. 1995;32 982-986.

[8] Mallbris L, Granath F, Hamsten A, Stahle M. Psoriasis is associated with lipid abnormalities at the onset of skin disease. Journal of American Academy of Dermatology. 2006;54 614-624.

[9] Eaglstein WH, Callen JP. Dermatologic comorbidities of diabetes mellitus and related issues. Archives of Dermatology. 2009;145 467-469.

[10] Gissondi P, Tessari G, Piaserico S, Schianchi S, Peserico A, Giannetti A. Prevalence of metabolic syndrome in patients with psoriasis: A hospital based case control study. British Journal of Dermatology. 2007;1 68-73.

[11] Nieman AL, Shin DB, Wang X, Margolis DJ, Troxel AB Gelfland JM. Prevalence of cardiovascular risk factors in patients with psoriasis. Journal of American Academy of Dermatology. 2006;10:829-35.

[12] Malbris L, Akre O, Granath F. Metabolic disorders in patients with psoriasis and psoriatic arthritis. Current Rheumatology Reports. 2006;8:355-63.

[13] Baumann H, Gauldie J. The acute phase response. Immunology Today. 1994;2 81-88.

[14] Rocha Pereire P. The inflammatory response in mild and severe psoriasis. British Journal of Dermatology. 2004;150 917-928.

[15] Ridker PM. C-reactive protein and other markers of inflammation in the prediction of cardiovascular disease in women. New England Journal of Medicine. 2000;342 836-883.

[16] Rohde LE, Hennekens CH, Ridker PM. Survey of C-reactive protein and cardiovascular risk factors in apparently healthy men. American Journal of Cardiology. 1999;84 1028-1032.

[17] Blake GJ, Ridker PM. Novel clinical markers of vascular wall inflammation. Circulation Research. 2001;89 763-771.

[18] Choudhury RP, Leyva F. C-Reactive protein, serum amyloid A protein and coronary events. Circulation. 1999;100 65-66.

[19] Steel DM, Whitehead AS. The major acute phase reactants: C reactive protein, serum amyloid P component and serum amyloid A protein. Immunology Today. 1994;2 81-88.

[20] Choudhury RP, Leyva F. C-Reactive protein, serum amyloid A protein and coronary events. Circulation. 1999;100 65-66.

[21] Jousilahti P, Salomaa V. The association of C-reactive protein, serum amyloid A and fibrinogen with prevalent coronary heart disease-baseline findings of the PAIS project. Atherosclerosis. 2001;156 451-456.

[22] Harb TS. Association of C-reactive protein and serum amyloid A with recurrent coronary events in stable patients after healing of acute myocardial infarction. American Journal of Cardiology. 2002;89 216-221.

[23] Mezaki T, Matsubara T. Plasma levels of soluble thrombomodulin, C-reactive protein and serum amyloid A protein in the atherosclerotic coronary circulation. Jpn Heart J. 2003; 44 601-612.

[24] Koenig W, Sund M. C-Reactive protein, a sensitive marker of inflammation, predicts future risk of coronary heart disease in initially healthy middle-aged men: results from the MONICA (Monitoring Trends and Determinants in Cardiovascular Disease) Augsburg Cohort Study, 1984 to 1992. Circulation 1999;99 237-242.

[25] Seideman P. Better effect of methotrexate on C-reactive protein during daily compared to weekly treatment in rheumatoid arthritis. Clinics in Rheumatology. 1993;12 210-213.

[26] Lan JL, Chou SJ, Chen DY, Chen YH, Hsieh TY, Young M. A comparative study of etanercept plus methotrexate and methotrexate alone in Taiwanese patients with active psoriatic arthritis: a 12-week, double-blind, randomized, placebo-controlled study. Journal of Formos Medical Association. 2004;103:618-23.

[27] Prodanovich S, Ma F, Taylor JR, Pezon C, Fasihi T, Kirsner RS. Methotrexate reduces incidence of vascular diseases in veterans with psoriasis or rheumatoid arthritis. Journal of American Academy of Dermatology. 2005;52(2) 262-267.

[28] Spadaro A, Riccieri V. Comparison of cyclosporin A and methotrexate in the treatment of psoriatic arthritis: A one-year prospective study. Clinical Experimental Rheumatology. 1995;13 589-593.

[29] Ohtsuka T. The correlation between response to oral cyclosporin therapy and systemic inflammation, metabolic abnormality in patients with psoriasis. Archives of Dermatological Research. 2008;300 545-550.

[30] Strober B, Teller C. Effects of etanercept on C-reactive protein levels in psoriasis and psoriatic arthritis. British Journal of Dermatology. 2008;159 322-330.

[31] Buch MH, Seto Y. C-reactive protein as a predictor of infliximab treatment outcome in patients with rheumatoid arthritis: Defining subtypes of nonresponse and subsequent response to etanercept. Arthritis Rheumotolgy. 2005;52 42-48.

[32] Ryan C, Leonardi CL, Krueger JG, Kimball AB, Strober BE, Gordon KB, Langley RG, de Lemos JA, Daoud Y, Blankenship D, Kazi S, Kaplan DH, Friedewald VE, Menter A. Association between biologic therapies for chronic plaque psoriasis and cardiovascular events: a meta-analysis of randomized controlled trials. JAMA. 2011 24;306(8) 864-871.

[33] Ramadori G, Sipe JD, Dinarello CA, Mixel SB, Colten HR. Pretranslational modulation of acute phase hepatic protein synthesis by murine recombinant IL-1 and purified human IL-1. Journal of Experimental Medicine. 1985;162 930-942.

[34] Thorn CF, Lu ZY, Whitehead AS. Regulation of the human acute phase by serum amyloid A genes by tumour necrosis factor-α, interleukin-6 and glucocorticoids in hepatic and epithelial cell lines. Scandinavian Journal of Immunology. 2004;59 152-158.

[35] Moshage HJ, Roelofs HMJ, Van Pelt JF, Hazenberg BPC, Van Lecuwen MA, Limburg PC et al. The effect of interleukin-1, interlekin-6 and its relationship on the synthesis of serum amyloid A and C-reactive protein in primary cultures of adult human hepatocytes. Bichemstry Biophysics Research Community. 1988;155 112-117.

[36] Brinckerhoff CE, Mitchell TI, Karmilowicz MJ, Kluve B, Benson MD. Autocrine induction of collegenase by serum amyloid A-like and β2microglobulin-like proteins. Science. 1989;243 655-657.

[37] Johnson BD. Serum amyloid A as a predictor of coronary artery disease and cardiovascular outcome in women: the National Heart, Lung and Blood Institute-Sponsored Women's Ischemia Syndrome Evaluation (WISE). Circulation. 2004;109 726-732.

[38] Jousilahti P, Salomaa V. The association of C-reactive protein, serum amyloid A and fibrinogen with prevalent coronary heart disease-baseline findings of the PAIS project. Atherosclerosis. 2001;156 451-456.

[39] Dogan S, Atakan N. Is serum amyloid A protein a better indicator of inflammation in severe psoriasis? British Journal of Dermatol. 2010; 163 875-89.

[40] Tamagawa-Mineoka R, Katoh N, Kishimoto S. Platelet activation in patients with psoriasis: Increased plasma levels of platelet-derived microparticles and soluble P-selectin. Journal of the American Academy of Dermatology. 2010;62 621-626.

[41] Kaur S, Zilmer K, Leping V, Zilmer M. The levels of adiponectin and leptin and their relation to other markers of cardiovascular risk in patients with psoriasis. Journal of the European Academy of Dermatology and Venerology. 2011, 25, 1328–1333.

[42] Kanelleas A, Liapi C, Katoulis A, Stavropoulos P, Avgerinou G, Georgala S, Economopoulos T, Stavrianeas NG, Katsambas A. The role of inflammatory markers in assessing disease severity and response to treatment in patients with psoriasis treated with etanercept. Clinical Experimental Dermatology. 2011;36(8) 845-850.

[43] Kamata M, Tada Y, Tatsuta A, Kawashima T, Shibata S, Mitsui H, Asano Y, Sugaya M, Kadono T, Kanda N, Watanabe S, Sato S. Serum lipocalin-2 levels are increased in patients with psoriasis. Clinical Experimental Dermatology. 2012 ;37(3) 296-299.

[44] Xydakis AM, Case CC, Jones PH. Adiponectin, inflammation and the expression of the metabolic syndrome in obese individuals: The impact of rapid weight loss through caloric restriction. Journal of Clinical Endocrinololgy Metabolism. 2004;89 2697-2703.

[45] Bruun JM, Verdich C, Toubro S, Artrup A, Richelsen B. Association between measures of insulin sensitivity and circulating levels of interleukin-8, interleukin-6 and tumor necrosis factor-α. Effect of weight loss in obese men. Eur Journal of Endocrinology. 2003;148 535-542.

[46] Hamminga EA, Van der Lely AJ, Neumann HAM, Thio HB. Chronic inflammation in psoriasis and obesity: Implications for therapy. Medical Hypotheses. 2006;67 768-773.

[47] Sterry W, Strober BE, Menter A. Obesity in psoriasis: the metabolic, clinical and therapeutic implications. Report of an interdisciplinary conference and review. British Journal of Dermatology. 2007;157 649–655.

http://dx.doi.org/10.5772/54347

[48] Sommer DM, Jenisch S, Suchan M, Christophers E, Weichenthal M. Increased prevalence of the metabolic syndrome in patients with moderate to severe psoriasis. Archives of Dermatological Research 2006; 298 321–328.

[49] Augustin M, Glaeske G, Radtke MA, Christophers E, Reich K, Schafer I. Epidemiology and comorbidity of psoriasis in children. British Journal of Dermatologyl. 2010;162 633-636.

[50] Koebnick C, Black MH, Smith N, Der-Sarkissian JK, Porter AH, Jacobsen SJ, et al. The association of psoriasis and elevated blood lipids in overweight and obese children. J Pediatr 2011; 159 577-583.

[51] Au S, Goldminz M, Loo DS, Dumont N,a Levine D, Volf E et al. Association between pediatric psoriasis and the metabolic syndrome. Journal of the American Academy of Dermatology. 2012; 66 1012-1013.

[52] Friedewald VE, Cather JC, Gordon KB, Kavanaugh A, Ridker PM, Roberts WC. The Editor's Roundtable: Psoriasis, Inflammation, and Coronary Artery Disease. The American Journal of Cardiology. 2007;

[53] Friedewald VE, Cather JC Gelfand J, Gordon KBGibbons GH, Grundy SM, Jarratt MT et al. AJC Editor's Consensus: Psoriasis and Coronary Artery Disease. The American Journal of Cardiology. 2008;102 1631–1643.

[54] Ahlehoff O, Gislason GH, Jørgensen CH, Lindhardsen J, Charlot M, Olesen JB, Abildstrøm SZ, Skov L, Torp-Pedersen C, Hansen PR. Psoriasis and risk of atrial fibrillation and ischaemic stroke: a Danish Nationwide Cohort Study. European Heart Journal. 2012;33(16): 2054-2064.

[55] Mehta N, Yiding Y, Pinnelas R, Krishnamoorthy P, Shin DB, Troxel AB, Gelfand JM. Attributable Risk Estimate of Severe Psoriasis on Major Cardiovascular Events. Am J Med. 2011 August ; 124(8): 775.

[56] Gelfand JM, Neimann AL, Shin DB, Wang X, Margolis DJ, Troxel B. Risk of myocardial infarction in patients with psoriasis. JAMA 2006;296:1735–1741.

[57] Kural BV, Örem A, Cimsit G, Uydu HA, Yandi YE, Alver A. Plasma homocysteine and its relationships with atherothrombotic markers in psoriatic patients. Clinica Chim Acta. 2003;332 23-30.

Section 3

Treatment of Psoriasis

Chapter 6

Treatment of Psoriasis with Topical Agents

Robyn S. Fallen, Anupam Mitra,
Laura Morrissey Rogers and Hermenio Lima

Additional information is available at the end of the chapter

http://dx.doi.org/10.5772/53759

1. Introduction

The history of immunosuppressive drugs is linked to both the evolution of scientific understanding of inflammatory diseases and the development of organ allografts. These drugs are part of a valuable arsenal for the treatment of diseases mediated by the immune system. As medical and public health practices have evolved, infectious processes are no longer the primary diagnostic and therapeutic challenge posed by dermatological conditions. Emerging in this void are cutaneous manifestations mediated by the immune system that present new management issues and require extensive use of the group of drugs described as immunomodulating agents. Psoriasis, among many other diseases in the purview of the dermatologist, is treated with these medications. Observing the use of these medications also helps to illustrate the evolution of dermatologic therapeutics. Some of these drugs, such as topical corticosteroids, are considered the basis of the dermatological therapeutic arsenal. To use these medications appropriately, it is important to be aware of both facts and myths concerning the action of immunosuppressive agents and the burden of side effects. [1]

The objective of this chapter is to discuss some characteristics of modern immunomodulators that are still useful for psoriasis treatment in the biological era. Moreover, it aims to dispel myths that might have a negative impact on the use of such drugs by clinicians. The primary focus is on immunomodulators that have been successfully used in the treatment of psoriasis. As such, several aspects of psoriasis immunopathophysiology and regulatory pathways of immune cells are explored [2]. Furthermore, it is likely that there is a considerable amount of similarity in concepts within this class of medications, given that these mechanisms describe immunomodulator drugs. Within this framework, the intention is to provide important insight into how the immune system can be modulated by these drugs used to treat psoriasis in a more traditional fashion.

2. Clinical manifestation of psoriasis

Psoriasis is a chronic, inflammatory, multi-system disorder characterized by abnormal epidermal differentiation and hyperproliferation thought to be related to abnormal immune system activity. According to data from various resources, about 2-3% of the general population suffers from psoriasis. Accepting and extrapolating these rates globally, approximately 140 to 210 million people live with psoriasis Although psoriasis is usually benign, it is a lifelong illness with remissions and exacerbations and is sometimes refractory to treatment. Nonetheless, the majority of the cases are mild or moderate psoriasis [3]. A recent study observed 75.8% of patients to have a psoriasis area severity index (PASI) of <20 [4]. Moreover, 17-55% of patients experience remissions of varying lengths. Plaque-type psoriasis is the most common form, affecting 80 – 90% of patients. Inverse, erythrodermic, pustular and guttate forms of psoriasis have also been described. Patients present with sharply demarcated, erythematous plaques covered by silvery white scales, most commonly on the extensor surfaces and the scalp. The natural history is variable but is often chronic and relapsing, and patients may experience extracutaneous manifestations commonly including nail involvement and psoriatic arthritis in up to 20% of patients [5].

3. Psoriasis pathogenesis

In the context of a complex multifactorial genetic background, environmental stimuli, such as bacterial antigens, act agonistically on Toll-like receptors (TLR) on the surface of keratinocytes (KC). In psoriatic patients, this stimulus induces the production of several inflammatory mediators by KC that are released to the adjacent underlying dermis. In this pro-inflammatory environment, endothelial cells from small vessels start to express adhesion molecules, such as intracellular adhesion molecule-1 (ICAM-1 or CD54), vascular cell adhesion molecule-1 (VCAM-1, or CD106), and E-selectin (CD62E). These superficial molecular modifications allow leukocytes and lymphocytes to migrate to the dermis, attracted by inflammatory chemokines released by KC. Macrophage inflammatory protein-3 A (MIP3A), produced by the keratinocytes, binds to its receptor CCR6 on leukocyte surface, blocks the leukocyte migration, and induces the formation of structure lymphoid tissues in the dermis. The CD11c+ plasmacytoid dendritic cells (DC) and CD3+ T cells in the organized lymphoid tissue initiate a process of cross communication based on cytokine production.

The activated DC (CD11c+) produces TNF-α, IL-12, IL-20 and IL-23. CD3+ T cells in response to IL-12, initially produce IFN-γ and are considered Th1 (Phase I of the cytokine pathway). Later in the process, the continuous activation of KC induces the presence of transforming growth factor (TGF)-β in the field. In the presence of IL-23 and TGF-β, the IL-12 chronic stimulated CD3+ Th1 cells evolve into Th17 CD3+ T cells (Phase II of the cytokine pathway). Th17 cells produce IL-17 and IL-22. IL-17 and IL-22 act in synergy with IL-19, IL-20 and IL-24, produced by IL-20-activated resident macrophages, to induce keratinocyte activation and proliferation (Phase III of the cytokine pathway). The activated and proliferative keratinocytes

http://dx.doi.org/10.5772/53759

produce other proinflammatory cytokines, which maintain the vicious inflammatory cycle of plaque psoriasis. Among the proinflammatory cytokines is IL-8 (recently converted to CXCL8), is related to the migration of neutrophils to the plaque in psoriasis. Growth-regulated oncogene (GRO)-α, also known as CXCL1, predisposes tissues to further cellular proliferation. Human beta defensin (HBD)-2, HBD-3, and LL-37 induce microbacterial destruction and the release of further bacterial antigens to the immunological environment.

4. Immunomodulators – Basic concept of drugs used to treat psoriasis

In a homeostatic situation, the immune system interacts with many antigens without notice in a healthy individual [6]. However, the development of a hypersensitivity response induced by the chronic stimulation of the immune system results in the clinical manifestation of a specific group of illnesses [7]. The lack of control of the immune response is the basis of the clinical manifestation of these diseases. In the majority of these cases, there is an increase in the immune response activity. Therefore, the manifestation of a hypersensitivity reaction induces the pathogenesis of autoimmune and other inflammatory diseases [8].

The basic approach for treatment of these illnesses is manipulating the immune system to reduce its activity. In these cases, the therapeutic goal is fine-tuning of the milieu to downgrade the pathological response and return the immune system to a state of controlled homeostasis [9, 10]. However, the modulation of the system has to bring the balance to its normal limits without reducing it beyond these boundaries. It can be compared to adjusting the volume and the tone of music in an orchestra. High volume and distortions reduce the beauty of the music and can cause discomfort. In adjusting the volume and correcting the distortions, the maestro modulates the music, creating a pleasant sensation while still ensuring that each component remains audible.

Medications for treatment of autoimmune diseases modulate the immune system [11]. They do not cause immunosuppression because they treat a hyper-activated system [12]. Rather, they bring the immune system to its normal levels (Figure 1).

Bringing the immune system to its normal levels resolves the symptoms caused by the overactive inflammatory response. Immunosuppression occurs only when the immune system is reduced to a level below its physiological level by these drugs [13]. Therefore, the correct use of the various immunomodulators intends to bring the patient to a controlled homeostasis with an absence of symptoms.

4.1. Development of the actual recommendations for treatment of psoriasis

There has been considerable debate in the literature regarding the most appropriate method to determine the initial treatment in psoriasis. The general observation of the psoriasis guideline therapy reveals that the basic decisions are based on psoriasis intensity and its form of clinical manifestation. Body Surface Area (BSA) and Psoriasis Area and Severity Index (PASI) are the main criteria to decide therapeutic strategy in psoriasis.

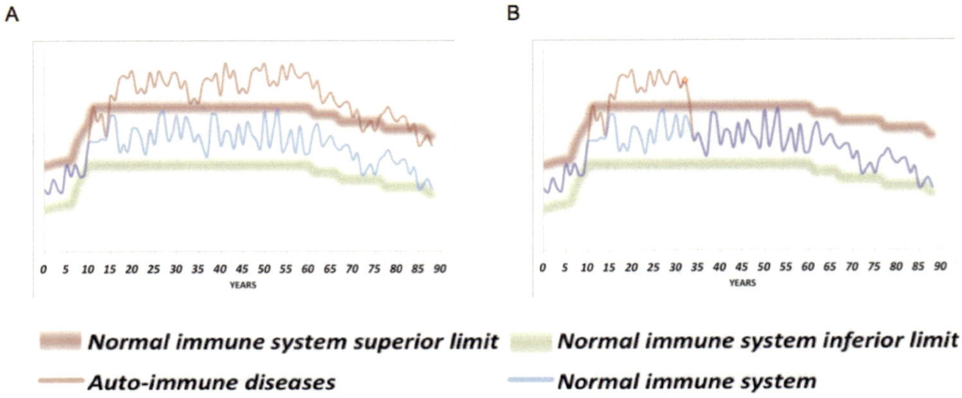

Figure 1. Schematic representation of immune system activity and its limits over the life-course. The blue line shows the immune system action within the normal limits boundaries. The red line displays the hyper-activated portion of the system immune activity that creates the autoimmune disease. A. It expresses a patient with untreated autoimmune disease. B. It illustrates a patient treated with a successful immunomodulator (orange diamond). The immunomodulator brings the immune system within normal immune system limits and not cause immunosuppression.

It is well accepted that a BSA higher than 10% and/ or a PASI higher than 10 is the limit that determines the use of systemic medication (Figure 2) [14]. This elementary principle is found on the balance between risk and benefits of any therapy. The use of this guideline generally results in a ration and effective therapy for psoriatic patients; however, it is not an absolute rule. These therapy guideline suggestions are best paired with a recommended route of administration and should always be mediated by the good judgement of an analytical physician.

Therapy decisions and guidelines for psoriasis treatment have historically been based on clinical trials and empirical experience with available medications. Historical review implies a tendency of an inverse order between pathophysiology understanding and psoriasis treatment. The understanding of psoriasis pathophysiology was not the basis of drug treatment development in the majority of the cases. Studies in other fields, or pure empirical

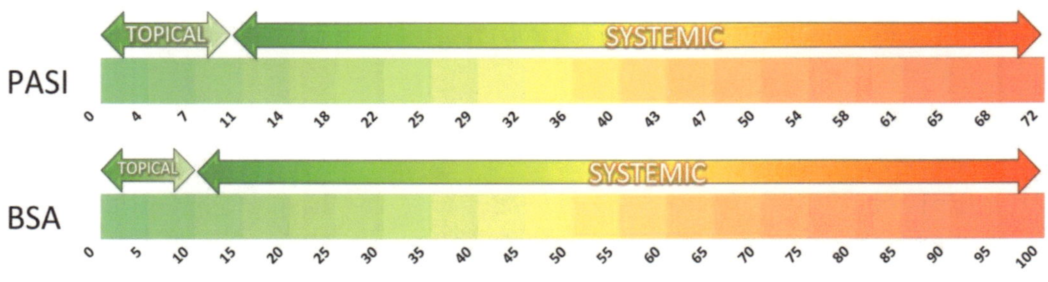

Figure 2. PASI and BSA scales. The putative limit between the use of topical and systemic treatment for psoriasis are demonstrated in both ribbons.

observation, resulted in the use of immunomodulators for psoriasis. The effective use of some of these drugs resulted in the actual immunopathophysiology model of psoriasis, not the other way around. For example, the etiology of psoriasis was once described as primarily and essentially an epidermal problem, independent of immunologic phenomena [15]. The main objective of cytotoxic drugs developed in the 20th century, such as methotrexate, was to reduce keratinocyte proliferation. However, immunological studies on psoriatic patients identified changes in humoral immune response as part of the overall problem but not the cause [16, 17]. The efficacy of cytotoxic drugs in the late 1960s paved the road for ideas about the role of the immune system in psoriasis [18, 19]. Further investigations in the 1970s revealed the role of immunologic factors in psoriasis. Here, these historical developments will be used as a context for the most recent guidelines in treatment of psoriasis.

4.2. Classification of the immunomodulators

To understand the drugs used in the treatment of psoriasis, the novice interested in this subject ought to know how these mediations are classified. Drugs that modulate the immune system can be classified as modifiers of the immune response to a specific antigen or antigens, nonspecific modulators, and agents that affect the inflammatory response. They can also be used in topical and systemic forms.

Antigen specific immune modifiers affect different stages of immune response. An example of this process is the use of anti-Rh antibodies. The desensitization to allergen is another example of antigen-specific immunosuppression.

Drugs such as cyclophosphamide, azathioprine, methotrexate and chlorambucil are the prototype of nonspecific antigen modulators. These drugs derive their immunomodulatory function primarily through cytotoxicity to immune effector cells. They are used in the treatment of both autoimmune and neoplastic diseases as well as in the control of rejection after organ and tissue transplantation. The medical field of transplantation has increased the use and development of these drugs. Another group of non antigen specific modulators inhibit the stimulation of T lymphocytes. They do so by inhibiting the T lymphocyte activation medicated by IL-2 and IL-2 receptors. Consequently, by inhibiting the activation of T lymphocytes these drugs reduce immune system activity. They include cyclosporine, tacrolimus, pimecrolimus and rapamycin.

Immunomudulators are also inhibitors of inflammatory response. Inflammation is the major manifestation of hyper-activation of the immune system. Thus, drugs that suppress the inflammatory response, such as NSAIDs and corticosteroids, can be useful in some circumstances.

5. Topical immunomodulators used in psoriasis

There continues to be significant evolution in psoriasis therapy in recent years. However, it is not surprising that topical forms of therapy are more prescribed than systemic forms in the treatment of psoriasis. Although psoriasis is usually benign, it is a lifelong illness with remissions and exacerbations and is sometimes refractory to treatment. Nonetheless, the majority of the cases of psoriasis are mild or moderate in severity [3] and can be effectively treated with topical immunomodulators. Some studies suggest that approximately 10% of patients with psoriasis progress to develop psoriatic arthritis. The systemic therapies are used in severe forms of psoriasis.

Topical therapy for psoriasis is used as the first form of treatment. The main objective of the therapy is to achieve short-term suppression of symptoms, and long-term modulation of disease severity. Moreover, topical therapy intends to improve quality of life with minimal adverse effects; however, there is no clear guidelines regarding the topical agent to be used in each type of psoriasis Therefore, the topical medications will be presented here on the basis of their historical evolution (Figure 3). There are some basic rules, which practitioners can apply in assessing when psoriasis can be managed with topical agents alone'. For example, patients with limited disease (usually < 10% of their body surface) can often be managed topically. For plaques, medium- to high-potency corticosteroids used daily is commonly the first choice of therapy. Coal tar preparations can be best used along with topical corticosteroids in rotation. Anthralin is more commonly used in short- term management of chronic plaque psoriasis. Vitamin D3 analogs are an effective treatment for mild to moderately severe plaque psoriasis and are well tolerated on the face and intertriginous areas without the use of corticosteroids.

5.1. Emollients

Emollient creams and lotions were developed because they are helpful in controlling scales and relieving pruritus. Emollients containing ingredients such as mineral oil are particularly helpful at relieving the dryness experienced with psoriasis. Emollients fill cavities and fissures of the skin with fat resulting in moisture retention and soft skin [20].

5.1.1. Emollients: Evidence summary for psoriasis treatment

They are available as over-the-counter preparations and should be applied at least once a day, preferably twice a day, but can be applied more often if required. Although both preparations are effective, most patients prefer creams to ointments, and compliance tends to be better with cream preparations.

5.2. Coal tar

Coal Tar was one of the first topical immunomodulators used for psoriasis treatment. One of the earliest references to its use was by the British Hospital for Diseases of the Skin in 1884. [21] Coal tar preparations can be effective for long-term management of psoriasis, with less side effects and rebound upon cessation than topical steroids. However, the exact mechanism of action of coal tar is not completely understood. The possible mechanism of action is the reduction of mitotic rate in the epidermis. This results in keratoplastic and anti-acanthotic properties. It can have an atrophogenic effect on the human epidermis. Finally, it has a photosensitizing effect with an absorption spectrum of 330–550 nm. This last effect is greatly

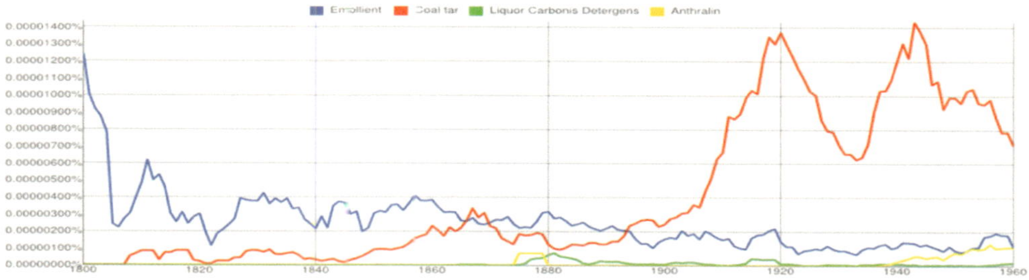

Figure 3. Google Books Ngram Viewer for old topical therapy for psoriasis. It displays a time line of how often the word Emollient, Coal tar, Liquor Carbonis Detergens, and Anthralin have occurred in a corpus of books written in English between 1800 and 1960. It roughly indicates the time of these therapies introduction in medicine.

enhanced by irradiation of the treated skin with UVA but not with UVB or UVC [22]. It seems that coal tar does not have a specific effect on the immune system of the skin [23].

When crude coal tar is refined or separate in different extracts, the result compound is called brown tar or liquor carbonis detergens (LCD). It is available in many different formulas such as soaks and shampoos. LCD is less effective than coal tar when combined with UVB for psoriasis therapy [24].

5.2.1. Coal tar: Evidence summary for psoriasis treatment

Tar preparations were once a popular treatment for psoriasis but have largely been replaced by topical corticosteroids due to the fact that these preparations are messy to use, can stain clothes, and have an unpleasant odor. They are effective in treating mild to moderate psoriasis [25].

5.3. Anthralin

Anthralin was developed from an herbal medication called Goa powder made from the bark of the South American araroba tree. Anthralin can be compounded in various vehicles and strengths, from 0.1% up to 10% or higher when specially compounded. It is usually necessary to add 3 to 10% salicylic acid in the formulation, not only as a keratolytic but also as a preservative to retard the oxidation of anthralin. Anthralin also causes a brown–red discoloration of the skin [26].

It is moderately effective and quite safe in plaque psoriasis. As for the main mechanism of action in psoriasis, anthralin is known to have antimitotic activity. The major side effect is occasional irritation. Use on acute, exudative, inflamed psoriatic plaques should be prevented. Irritation is more likely to occur in the perilesional skin than on the psoriasis plaque. Short contact treatment is used to reduce irritation but application for 8–12 hours is more effective [27]. The combination of the anthralin compound and UVB phototherapy is known as the Ingram regimen [28].

5.3.1. Anthralin: Evidence summary for psoriasis treatment

Anthralin used to be a mainstay for the topical treatment of psoriasis in the inpatient setting. However, its use has declined because of the availability of alternatives. It has been reported to be successful in treating mild to moderate psoriasis. When using Anthralin, it is best to start at the lowest strength and increase gradually as required according to response. Adverse effects include severe skin irritation, staining of clothing, and unpleasant smell.

5.4. Topical steroids

Topical steroids are the most used medication in the treatment of psoriasis. Corticosteroids were discovered in 1935 as compound E or cortisone [29]. The first therapeutic uses were in the treatment of rheumatoid arthritis and rheumatic fever followed by the treatment of inflammatory skin disease [30]. The topical use of steroids originated in 1952 as compound F or hydrocortisone [31]. Finally, psoriasis was included in the list of skin diseases treatable with hydrocortisone in 1955 [32].

The next step in the development of topical steroids included numerous modifications of the molecule and improvements in delivery systems of the drugs to increase their anti-inflammatory activity. Application of a thin film to psoriatic plaques two to three times daily is the basic instruction of topical steroids usage. Topical steroids have different potencies based on their formulations [33]. The efficacy is directly related to the skin penetration of steroid molecules and the rate of absorption is influenced by the steroid chemical structure. Other factors such as formulation vehicle and status of the skin also play a role in the absorption of the medication [34, 35].

It is not an easy decision to prescribe topical steroid for psoriasis. Among many other factors, anatomical site, amount, frequency of application should be considered too' [36]. For example, no topical corticosteroids should be used on the face, axilla, or groin, other than low-potency ones, unless otherwise recommended by the doctor. These concerns are related to the action of corticosteroids on the epidermis, which is to reduce the epidermis' ability to proliferate by interfering with RNA synthesis. Steroid antimitotic effect in cutaneous psoriasis demonstrates that the therapeutic effects are under the stratum corneum [33, 37].

Steroid antimitotic effects on the skin can cause a thinning of the epidermis. This can occur within 7 days of use of high dose topical steroids. All layers of the epidermis are reduced in thickness by 3 weeks of strong topical steroid use. The thinning of the epidermis impairs physiological functions of the epidermis and may be associated with the rebound of inflammation, which is a paradoxical effect. Thus, potent topical glucocorticosteroids will cause anti-inflammatory effects when first applied but with subsequent applications their therapeutic action rapidly diminishes, which is known as tachyphylaxis [38]. However, after a rest period of a few days, the same initial beneficial response may be produced again, but this will also disappear if the steroid is again continued topically. Therefore, steroids should be used for 2 to 3 weeks and then tapered with the intention of discontinuing the use of the steroid cream [39].

Effect of topical steroid action is not limited to the epidermis as they are able to penetrate the stratum corneum and are absorbed into both the epidermis and the dermis. Reduction of dermis volume occurs within 1-3 weeks of using high dose topical steroids. This acute effect also results from interference of RNA synthesis in fibroblasts' [40]. These cells do not produce primarily hyaluronic acid, which decreases dermal water content. However, the chronic use causes abnormal synthesis of collagen and elastin that is the cause of dermal atrophy and impaired wound healing [41, 42].

The steroid molecules are also absorbed to some degree into circulation when they reach the dermis. The absorption in large areas of skin after chronic use may be sufficient to cause systemic effects such as adrenocortical suppression. Therefore, systemic side effects have become a very real concern with the use potent topical steroids [43]. This is one of the most important criteria for use of BSA or PASI 10 to initiate systemic medication. Although it is rare to see clinical systemic effects in an adult patient, there have been reported cases of hypothalamic-pituitary-adrenal (HPA) axis suppression, Cushing's syndrome, cataracts, and glaucoma. Moreover, children are more at risk for systemic side effects because they have greater body mass to body surface ratio than adults. In general, high dose super potent topical steroids are not recommended for children under age 12 because they can cause growth retardation and failure to thrive [44, 45].

As immunomodulators, steroids initiate their mechanisms of action by binding to intracellular receptors, and inhibits protein synthesis resulting in immunosuppression. The majority of these events occur at the dermis. Steroids effect cell trafficking since they reduce the expression of adhesion molecules on the vascular endothelium. Corticosteroids also have functional effects. They alter the release of neutrophil lysosomal enzymes, decrease production of IL-1 by monocytes, induce reduction of IL-2 by T lymphocytes, and interfere with macrophage antigen presentation. Corticosteroids reduce the binding of immunoglobulin Fc and C3b receptors. They block lymphocyte proliferation and reduce delayed hypersensitivity responses. Many other effects are observed with corticosteroids, but these are considered to be the most important [44, 46].

5.4.1. Topical steroids: Evidence summary for psoriasis treatment

One systematic review of topical corticosteroid preparations versus placebo for psoriasis clearly indicated that all corticosteroids performed better than placebo. The same study showed that potent corticosteroids had smaller benefits than very potent corticosteroids [47]. Therefore, with this in mind, pharmacological treatment of psoriasis should begin with the use of topical corticosteroids. They are easy to apply and suitable for combination with other therapies where monotherapy is insufficient. Generally, the lowest potency of topical corticosteroid should be used. Low-potency treatments are appropriate for lesions on the face or intertriginous areas or for infants. Adults mainly respond to a mid-potency agent. High-potency topical corticosteroids are usually reserved for adults requiring short-term treatment of thick plaques that are resistant to lower-potency agents [48].

5.5. Analogues of vitamin D3 for psoriasis

Calcipotriol, calcitriol and tacalcitol are analogues of vitamin D3. Calcitriol is the naturally occurring active form of vitamin D3. Keratinocytes possess receptors for 1,25-dihydroxyvitamin D. All vitamin D3 derivatives inhibit cell proliferation and stimulate differentiation of keratinocytes. These observations inspired the use of analogues of vitamin D3 for the treatment of psoriasis [49]. Vitamin D derivatives are more effective at improving psoriasis severity scores at 3 to 8 weeks when compared with placebo. However, the overall data has moderate-quality evidence [50].

Indicated for mild to moderately severe plaque psoriasis, there are more effects on the skin than simply the enhancement of epithelial cell differentiation. Calcitriol can modulate the skin's immune system through interfering with antigen presenting cells, regulatory T cell activation, cutaneous cytokine patterns, and adaptive immunity [52]. The final result is that vitamin D3 analogues effect inflammatory cell infiltration. Interestingly, like topical corticosteroids, tachyphylaxis can occur after a few weeks of use Vitamin D3 analogues. Therefore, rotational is a useful strategy to ensure maximum therapeutic benefit. This involves rotating vitamin D with other treatments every few weeks. Moreover, there is considerable evidence to suggest that the hyperproliferation and inflammatory components of the disease can be more rapidly controlled using mixtures of drugs such as the vitamin D3 analog calcipotriol and the steroid betamethasone dipropionate [53].

5.5.1. Analogues of vitamin D3: Evidence summary for psoriasis treatment

Vitamin D3 analogues have the advantage of being cosmetically more acceptable to patients than coal tar or anthralin preparations, but they may cause irritant dermatitis and photosensitivity in some patients. Calcitriol can be used on the scalp and flexural areas. Cream formulation may be well tolerated on the face and intertriginous areas. They should be avoided in generalised pustular erythrodermic exfoliative psoriasis and individuals with calcium metabolism disorders. Patients are limited to a maximum of 100 g/week because there is a potential risk of hypercalcemia and hypercalciuria, although this occurrence is rare.

5.6. Tazarotene

The use of oral retinoids for psoriasis treatment precedes that of their use topically. However, the success of these oral therapies, and the development of topical retinoids for other dermatoses, triggered the development of tazarotene. Tazarotene is a selective topical retinoid for psoriasis treatment. Efficacy and safety of this agent has been established as a monotherapy or in combination with other therapies, particularly topical corticosteroids and phototherapy [54, 55].

Like other retinoid derivatives, tazarotene binds the retinoic acid receptor (RAR) but in a class-specific manner. It preferentially binds to RAR-γ and RAR-β over RAR-α and it does not bind retinoid X receptor (RXR) [56]. As a result of the binding at the RAR receptor, tazarotene seems to cause a reduction in proliferation and normalizes the differentiation of keratinocytes [57]. It also possesses indirect anti-inflammatory properties by affecting keratinocyte chemokine production which reduces the dermal infiltration [58].

Tazarotene may be effective in the short term at improving symptoms of mild to moderate chronic plaque psoriasis [59]. It may cause skin irritation, including burning, stinging and itch in up to 30% of users [60]. It is potentially teratogenic and is contraindicated in women who may be/become pregnant [61, 62].

5.6.1. Tazarotene: Evidence summary for psoriasis treatment

Tazarotene may be effective as a short term therapy of mild to moderate chronic plaque psoriasis. It may cause skin irritation, including burning, stinging and itch in up to 30% of users. It is potentially teratogenic and is contraindicated pregnant or would be pregnant women'

5.7. Topical calcineurin inhibitors

Calcineurin inhibitors (CIs), such as tacrolimus and pimecrolimus, are large lipophilic molecules that may be used topically in the treatment of psoriasis [63]. Their lipophilicity and size keep them in the skin with minimal systemic absorption [64, 65]. The main advantage of these drugs is the possibility of maintenance therapy for long periods eliminating the need for prolonged corticosteroids and their side effects [66].

Tacrolimus and pimecrolimus interact intracellularly by inhibiting the protein NFAT activation (Nuclear Factor Activating T cell) by calcineurin [67]. This works by blocking T lymphocyte mediated signaling and cytokine production. Topical CIs prevent transcription of inflammatory cytokines, including interleukin (IL)-2, IL-3, IL-4, IL-5, interferon (IFN)-γ and tumor necrosis factor (TNF)-α, which normally contribute to psoriatic lesions [68]. Downregulation of the high-affinity IgE receptor on Langerhans cells and inhibition of the release of inflammatory mediators from mast cells and basophils may also partly explain the effect of CIs when used topically [69]. Finally, recent evidence suggests that topical CIs may not act primarily by inhibiting the calcineurin/NFAT axis in lymphocytes in the skin but rather that they may instead act by decreasing NFAT2 activity in follicular keratinocytes [70]. These characteristics further support the topical use of CIs in the treatment of psoriasis.

Currently, calcineurin inhibitors are approved for atopic dermatitis (AD) treatment only. Despite their efficacy in AD management, CIs are ineffective in non-intertriginous psoriatic plaques management. This lack of efficacy is credited to the inability of CIs to penetrate the thick psoriatic plaques, however, they may be effective when used under occlusion on descaled small plaques. Tacrolimus therapy is more effective in the treatment of the face and intertriginous areas and is particularly useful because it does not cause skin atrophy or changes in collagen synthesis [71].

Most studies about the safety of CIs are centered on patients with atopic dermatitis. However, these products continue to be used off-label for psoriasis. Topical adverse effects of CIs may actually occur less frequently on the thick plaques of psoriasis. Both topical tacrolimus and pimecrolimus may cause a stinging or burning sensation. Occasionally, patients using CIs experience flu-like symptoms, headaches, folliculitis and increased flushing after alcohol use. The FDA has raised concerns about the safety of CIs and has issued a black-box warning regarding the use of both tacrolimus and pimecrolimus. This concern is based on evidence of malignancy after long-term use of oral CIs and is not related to topical use. However, the FDA did not confirm a casual relationship between the use of CIs and the cases of malignancy. Further investigations regarding the safety of topical immunomodulators did not confirm the FDAs concerns. Furthermore, clinical evidence up to this point has not shown an enhanced risk of cancer after the use of either topical tacrolimus or pimecrolimus.

5.7.1. Calcineurin inhibitors: Evidence summary for psoriasis treatment

Calcineurin inhibitors have moderate efficacy for facial and inverse or intertriginous psoriasis. Their main indications are facial or inverse psoriasis that have not been responsive to weak or moderate strength topical steroids.

6. Summary of topical medications used in psoriasis treatment

Treatment of psoriasis depends on the type and severity of the disease. Typically, topical therapies are used to treat mild and localized psoriasis. Topical treatments are the foundation for mild to moderate psoriasis. However, this approach can decrease the number and thickness of the plaque lesions, and reduce the percentage of body surface involved. In general, pharmacological treatment should start with the use of topical corticosteroids [72].

The complete clearance of lesions is often not a realistic goal with topical therapy but eventually remission can be reached. Frustration related to medication efficacy expectations, poor cosmetic characteristics of topical preparations, time consumption, fear of side effects, and inconvenience were found to be the most important reasons patients chose to deviate from provider recommendations of topical therapy [73]. Studies suggest that adherence with topical treatment in psoriasis is poor. Research has shown that only 50% of topical agent applications prescribed by physicians are actually used [74].

Patients with chronic psoriasis may be candidates for topical therapy depending on their baseline severity. Topical treatments include creams, ointments, and lotions. The choice of formulation depends on the area affected. Physicians should also select formulations that will be acceptable to the patient [75]. There is a consensus that topical emollients and salicylic acid are effective as initial and adjunctive therapy for people with chronic plaque psoriasis, but it is unclear whether tars are effective [76].

6.1. Routine suggestions for classical mild and moderate plaque psoriasis

Topical high-potency corticosteroids may be used as first-line therapies for patients with mild plaque psoriasis. Low-potency treatments are appropriate for infants. Other appropriate first-line options include topical calcipotriol and calcipotriol/betamethasone dipropionate in

http://dx.doi.org/10.5772/53759

combination. Non-medicinal emollients, including creams, ointments, and lotions should be used in combination with the above agents to potentiate their effects and to help restore the natural barrier of the skin. For appropriate patients, tazarotene may be used, either alone or in combination with topical corticosteroids. Patients requiring ongoing treatment with topical agents containing high-potency corticosteroids should be monitored regularly for adverse effects and steroid-sparing concomitant treatments should be introduced. The rotation of a nonsteroidal topical agent following initial treatment is indicated.

6.2. Routine suggestions for facial, flexural, or genital areas

Topical treatment with calcineurin inhibitors (0.1% tacrolimus ointment or 1% pimecrolimus cream) should be used. Topical corticosteroids such as 0.1% betamethasone may be used on an occasional or intermittent basis. Mild- or moderate-potency corticosteroids may also be used on an occasional or intermittent basis to treat facial and genital psoriasis. In moderate to severe facial, flexural, and genital disease, stronger corticosteroids may be applied to address nonresponsive psoriasis or acute flares in these areas.

6.3. Routine suggestions for scalp psoriasis

Topical corticosteroids and calcipotriol are all appropriate topical treatments. Betamethasone dipropionate lotion, clobetasol propionate solution, betamethasone valerate solution, or calcipotriol solution are also possibilities. Calcipotriol/betamethasone dipropionate combination gel is a recently emerging therapy.

6.4. Routine suggestions for palmar--plantar disease

For mild and moderate manifestations, potent corticosteroid or vitamin D analogues with salicylic acid preparations should be used. For intense forms, high-potency corticosteroids with salicylic acid and urea preparations are the main choice of therapy.

7. Conclusion

The treatment of diseases involving the immune system has progressed in recent years with the introduction of new immunomodulators in clinical practice. These drugs act at different points in the immune response and may significantly alter the immune response of the patient, especially if combined. However, topical therapies continue to serve as the fundamental basis for any physician when dealing with psoriasis. Understanding the mechanism of action of these drugs is necessary for better management and proper application in situations where clinical challenges appear. Further research and development in the field of topical immunomodulators will hopefully result in the design of even more effective drugs, with increased specificity of action and fewer side effects.

Author details

Robyn S. Fallen[1], Anupam Mitra[2], Laura Morrissey Rogers[1] and Hermenio Lima[3*]

*Address all correspondence to: hlima@mcmaster.ca

1 Michael G. DeGroote School of Medicine, Waterloo Regional Campus, McMaster University, Canada

2 Dermatology, UC Davis School of Medicine, VA Medical Center, Sacramento, CA, USA

3 Division of Dermatology, Department of Medicine, Michael G. DeGroote School of Medicine, McMaster University, Ontario, Canada

References

[1] Lima HC, Kimball AB. Targeting IL-23: insights into the pathogenesis and the treatment of psoriasis. Indian J Dermatol. 2010 Apr-Jun;55(2):171-5.

[2] Maeda S, Hayami Y, Naniwa T, Ueda R. The Th17/IL-23 Axis and Natural Immunity in Psoriatic Arthritis. Int J Rheumatol. 2012;2012:539683.

[3] Berger K, Ehlken B, Kugland B, Augustin M. Cost-of-illness in patients with moderate and severe chronic psoriasis vulgaris in Germany. J Dtsch Dermatol Ges. 2005 Jul; 3(7):511-8.

[4] Gourraud PA, Le Gall C, Puzenat E, Aubin F, Ortonne JP, Paul CF. Why statistics matter: limited inter-rater agreement prevents using the psoriasis area and severity index as a unique determinant of therapeutic decision in psoriasis. J Invest Dermatol. 2012 Sep;132(9):2171-5.

[5] Lima XT, Abuabara K, Kimball AB, Lima HC. Briakinumab. Expert Opin Biol Ther. 2009 Aug;9(8):1107-13.

[6] Quattroni P, Exley RM, Tang CM. New insights into pathogen recognition. Expert Rev Anti Infect Ther. 2011 Aug;9(8):577-9.

[7] Mitra A, Fallen RS, Lima HC. Cytokine-Based Therapy in Psoriasis. Clin Rev Allergy Immunol. 2012 Mar 18.

[8] Oboki K, Ohno T, Kajiwara N, Arae K, Morita H, Ishii A, et al. IL-33 is a crucial amplifier of innate rather than acquired immunity. Proc Natl Acad Sci U S A. 2010 Oct 26;107(43):18581-6.

[9] Kriegel MA, Manson JE, Costenbader KH. Does vitamin D affect risk of developing autoimmune disease?: a systematic review. Semin Arthritis Rheum. 2011 Jun;40(6): 512-31 e8.

[10] Salgado A, Boveda JL, Monasterio J, Segura RM, Mourelle M, Gomez-Jimenez J, et al. Inflammatory mediators and their influence on haemostasis. Haemostasis. 1994 Mar-Apr;24(2):132-8.

[11] Buerger C, Richter B, Woth K, Salgo R, Malisiewicz B, Diehl S, et al. Interleukin-1beta Interferes with Epidermal Homeostasis through Induction of Insulin Resistance: Implications for Psoriasis Pathogenesis. J Invest Dermatol. 2012 Sep;132(9):2206-14.

[12] Ipaktchi K, Mattar A, Niederbichler AD, Hoesel LM, Vollmannshauser S, Hemmila MR, et al. Attenuating burn wound inflammatory signaling reduces systemic inflammation and acute lung injury. J Immunol. 2006 Dec 1;177(11):8065-71.

[13] Fallen RS, Terpstra CR, Lima HC. Immunotherapies in dermatologic disorders. Med Clin North Am. 2012 May;96(3):565-82, x-xi.

[14] Krueger GG, Feldman SR, Camisa C, Duvic M, Elder JT, Gottlieb AB, et al. Two considerations for patients with psoriasis and their clinicians: what defines mild, moderate, and severe psoriasis? What constitutes a clinically significant improvement when treating psoriasis? J Am Acad Dermatol. 2000 Aug;43(2 Pt 1):281-5.

[15] Ingram JT. The approach to psoriasis. Br Med J. 1953 Sep 12;2(4836):591-4.

[16] Aswaq M, Farber EM, Moreci AP, Raffel S. Immunologic reactions in psoriasis. Arch Dermatol. 1960 Nov;82:663-6.

[17] Harber LC, March C, Ovary Z. Lack of passive cutaneous anaphylaxis in psoriasis. Arch Dermatol. 1962 Jun;85:716-9.

[18] Harris CC. Malignancy during methotrexate and steroid therapy for psoriasis. Arch Dermatol. 1971 May;103(5):501-4.

[19] Landau J, Gross BG, Newcomer VD, Wright ET. Immunologic Response of Patients with Psoriasis. Arch Dermatol. 1965 Jun;91:607-10.

[20] Levi K, Kwan A, Rhines AS, Gorcea M, Moore DJ, Dauskardt RH. Emollient molecule effects on the drying stresses in human stratum corneum. Br J Dermatol. 2010 Oct;163(4):695-703.

[21] Squire AJB. The pharmacopoeia of the British Hospital for Diseases of the Skin, London. 3rd ed. London: J. & A. Churchill; 1884.

[22] Thami GP, Sarkar R. Coal tar: past, present and future. Clin Exp Dermatol. 2002 Mar; 27(2):99-103.

[23] Puttick LM, Johnson GD, Walker L. The epidermal Langerhans' cell population in psoriasis during topical coal tar therapy. Acta Derm Venereol. 1986;66(4):343-6.

[24] Johnson C, Edison B, Brouda I, Green B. A novel LCD (coal tar) solution for psoriasis does not discolor naturally light or color-processed hair in an exaggerated exposure test model. J Cosmet Dermatol. 2009 Sep;8(3):211-5.

[25] Smith CH, Jackson K, Chinn S, Angus K, Barker JN. A double blind, randomized, controlled clinical trial to assess the efficacy of a new coal tar preparation (Exorex) in the treatment of chronic, plaque type psoriasis. Clin Exp Dermatol. 2000 Nov;25(8): 580-3.

[26] Ashton RE, Andre P, Lowe NJ, Whitefield M. Anthralin: historical and current perspectives. J Am Acad Dermatol. 1983 Aug;9(2):173-92.

[27] Afifi T, de Gannes G, Huang C, Zhou Y. Topical therapies for psoriasis: evidence-based review. Can Fam Physician. 2005 Apr;51:519-25.

[28] De Bersaques J. A retrospective study of the inpatient treatment of psoriasis with dithranol. Dermatologica. 1987;175(2):64-8.

[29] Bishop PM. Compound E. Guys Hosp Gaz. 1949 Aug 13;63(1593):249-53.

[30] Carlisle JM. Cortisone (compound E); summary of its clinical uses. Br Med J. 1950 Sep 9;2(4679):590-5.

[31] Sulzberger MB, Witten VH. The effect of topically applied compound F in selected dermatoses. J Invest Dermatol. 1952 Aug;19(2):101-2.

[32] Rattner H. The status of corticosteroid therapy in dermatology. Calif Med. 1955 Nov; 83(5):331-5.

[33] Pels R, Sterry W, Lademann J. Clobetasol propionate--where, when, why? Drugs Today (Barc). 2008 Jul;44(7):547-57.

[34] Badilli U, Sen T, Tarimci N. Microparticulate based topical delivery system of clobetasol propionate. AAPS PharmSciTech. 2011 Sep;12(3):949-57.

[35] Stein L. Clinical studies of a new vehicle formulation for topical corticosteroids in the treatment of psoriasis. J Am Acad Dermatol. 2005 Jul;53(1 Suppl 1):S39-49.

[36] Pardasani AG, Feldman SR, Clark AR. Treatment of psoriasis: an algorithm-based approach for primary care physicians. Am Fam Physician. 2000 Feb 1;61(3):725-33, 36.

[37] Katz HI. Topical corticosteroids. Dermatol Clin. 1995 Oct;13(4):805-15.

[38] Feldman SR. Tachyphylaxis to topical corticosteroids: the more you use them, the less they work? Clin Dermatol. 2006 May-Jun;24(3):229-30; discussion 30.

[39] du Vivier A, Stoughton RB. Tachyphylaxis to the action of topically applied corticosteroids. Arch Dermatol. 1975 May;111(5):581-3.

[40] Lindschau C, Kirsch T, Klinge U, Kolkhof P, Peters I, Fiebeler A. Dehydroepiandrosterone-induced phosphorylation and translocation of FoxO1 depend on the mineralocorticoid receptor. Hypertension. 2011 Sep;58(3):471-8.

[41] Hall G, Phillips TJ. Estrogen and skin: the effects of estrogen, menopause, and hormone replacement therapy on the skin. J Am Acad Dermatol. 2005 Oct;53(4):555-68; quiz 69-72.

[42] Asboe-Hansen G. Influence of corticosteroids on connective tissue. Dermatologica. 1976;152 Suppl 1:127-32.

[43] Bruner CR, Feldman SR, Ventrapragada M, Fleischer AB, Jr. A systematic review of adverse effects associated with topical treatments for psoriasis. Dermatol Online J. 2003 Feb;9(1):2.

[44] Morley KW, Dinulos JG. Update on topical glucocorticoid use in children. Curr Opin Pediatr. 2012 Feb;24(1):121-8.

[45] van de Kerkhof PC, Murphy GM, Austad J, Ljungberg A, Cambazard F, Duvold LB. Psoriasis of the face and flexures. J Dermatolog Treat. 2007;18(6):351-60.

[46] Del Rosso J, Friedlander SF. Corticosteroids: options in the era of steroid-sparing therapy. J Am Acad Dermatol. 2005 Jul;53(1 Suppl 1):S50-8.

[47] Mason AR, Mason J, Cork M, Dooley G, Edwards G. Topical treatments for chronic plaque psoriasis. Cochrane Database Syst Rev. 2009(2):CD005028.

[48] Lebwohl M. A clinician's paradigm in the treatment of psoriasis. J Am Acad Dermatol. 2005 Jul;53(1 Suppl 1):S59-69.

[49] Holick MF, Smith E, Pincus S. Skin as the site of vitamin D synthesis and target tissue for 1,25-dihydroxyvitamin D3. Use of calcitriol (1,25-dihydroxyvitamin D3) for treatment of psoriasis. Arch Dermatol. 1987 Dec;123(12):1677-83a.

[50] Mason J, Mason AR, Cork MJ. Topical preparations for the treatment of psoriasis: a systematic review. Br J Dermatol. 2002 Mar;146(3):351-64.

[51] Morimoto S, Onishi T, Imanaka S, Yukawa H, Kozuka T, Kitano Y, et al. Topical administration of 1,25-dihydroxyvitamin D3 for psoriasis: report of five cases. Calcif Tissue Int. 1986 Feb;38(2):119-22.

[52] Cutolo M, Plebani M, Shoenfeld Y, Adorini L, Tincani A. Vitamin D endocrine system and the immune response in rheumatic diseases. Vitam Horm. 2011;86:327-51.

[53] Queille-Roussel C, Hoffmann V, Ganslandt C, Hansen KK. Comparison of the antipsoriatic effect and tolerability of calcipotriol-containing products in the treatment of psoriasis vulgaris using a modified psoriasis plaque test. Clin Drug Investig. 2012 Sep 1;32(9):613-9.

[54] Gollnick H, Menter A. Combination therapy with tazarotene plus a topical corticosteroid for the treatment of plaque psoriasis. Br J Dermatol. 1999 Apr;140 Suppl 54:18-23.

[55] Marks R. Clinical safety of tazarotene in the treatment of plaque psoriasis. J Am Acad Dermatol. 1997 Aug;37(2 Pt 3):S25-32.

[56] Chandraratna RA. Tazarotene--first of a new generation of receptor-selective retinoids. Br J Dermatol. 1996 Oct;135 Suppl 49:18-25.

[57] Nagpal S, Thacher SM, Patel S, Friant S, Malhotra M, Shafer J, et al. Negative regulation of two hyperproliferative keratinocyte differentiation markers by a retinoic acid receptor-specific retinoid: insight into the mechanism of retinoid action in psoriasis. Cell Growth Differ. 1996 Dec;7(12):1783-91.

[58] Wolf JE, Jr. Potential anti-inflammatory effects of topical retinoids and retinoid analogues. Adv Ther. 2002 May-Jun;19(3):109-18.

[59] van de Kerkhof PC, Kragballe K, Segaert S, Lebwohl M. Factors impacting the combination of topical corticosteroid therapies for psoriasis: perspectives from the International Psoriasis Council. J Eur Acad Dermatol Venereol. 2011 Oct;25(10):1130-9.

[60] Weinstein GD, Koo JY, Krueger GG, Lebwohl MG, Lowe NJ, Menter MA, et al. Tazarotene cream in the treatment of psoriasis: Two multicenter, double-blind, randomized, vehicle-controlled studies of the safety and efficacy of tazarotene creams 0.05% and 0.1% applied once daily for 12 weeks. J Am Acad Dermatol. 2003 May;48(5):760-7.

[61] Shapiro S, Heremans A, Mays DA, Martin AL, Hernandez-Medina M, Lanes S. Use of topical tretinoin and the development of noncutaneous adverse events: evidence from a systematic review of the literature. J Am Acad Dermatol. 2011 Dec;65(6): 1194-201.

[62] Duvic M. Pharmacologic profile of tazarotene. Cutis. 1998 Feb;61(2 Suppl):22-6.

[63] Bagan J, Compilato D, Paderni C, Panzarella V, Picciotti M, Lorenzini G, et al. Topical therapies for Oral Lichen Planus management and their efficacy: a narrative review. Curr Pharm Des. 2012 May 25.

[64] Wollina U, Hansel G, Koch A, Abdel-Naser MB. Topical pimecrolimus for skin disease other than atopic dermatitis. Expert Opin Pharmacother. 2006 Oct;7(14):1967-75.

[65] Nghiem P, Pearson G, Langley RG. Tacrolimus and pimecrolimus: from clever prokaryotes to inhibiting calcineurin and treating atopic dermatitis. J Am Acad Dermatol. 2002 Feb;46(2):228-41.

[66] Callen J, Chamlin S, Eichenfield LF, Ellis C, Girardi M, Goldfarb M, et al. A systematic review of the safety of topical therapies for atopic dermatitis. Br J Dermatol. 2007 Feb;156(2):203-21.

[67] Al-Daraji WI, Grant KR, Ryan K, Saxton A, Reynolds NJ. Localization of calcineurin/NFAT in human skin and psoriasis and inhibition of calcineurin/NFAT activation in human keratinocytes by cyclosporin A. J Invest Dermatol. 2002 May;118(5):779-88.

[68] Kantrow SP, Gierman JL, Jaligam VR, Zhang P, Piantadosi CA, Summer WR, et al. Regulation of tumor necrosis factor cytotoxicity by calcineurin. FEBS Lett. 2000 Oct 20;483(2-3):119-24.

[69] Marsland AM, Soundararajan S, Joseph K, Kaplan AP. Effects of calcineurin inhibitors on an in vitro assay for chronic urticaria. Clin Exp Allergy. 2005 May;35(5):554-9.

[70] Fiorentino DF, Chen RO, Stewart DB, Brown KK, Sundram UN. The direct cellular target of topically applied pimecrolimus may not be infiltrating lymphocytes. Br J Dermatol. 2011 May;164(5):996-1003.

[71] Brune A, Miller DW, Lin P, Cotrim-Russi D, Paller AS. Tacrolimus ointment is effective for psoriasis on the face and intertriginous areas in pediatric patients. Pediatr Dermatol. 2007 Jan-Feb;24(1):76-80.

[72] Nast A, Boehncke WH, Mrowietz U, Ockenfels HM, Philipp S, Reich K, et al. S3 - Guidelines on the treatment of psoriasis vulgaris (English version). Update. J Dtsch Dermatol Ges. 2012 Mar;10 Suppl 2:S1-95.

[73] Laws PM, Young HS. Topical treatment of psoriasis. Expert Opin Pharmacother. 2010 Aug;11(12):1999-2009.

[74] Devaux S, Castela A, Archier E, Gallini A, Joly P, Misery L, et al. Adherence to topical treatment in psoriasis: a systematic literature review. J Eur Acad Dermatol Venereol. 2012 May;26 Suppl 3:61-7.

[75] Hendriks AG, Keijsers RR, de Jong EM, Seyger MM, van de Kerkhof PC. Combinations of classical time-honoured topicals in plaque psoriasis: a systematic review. J Eur Acad Dermatol Venereol. 2012 Jul 11.

[76] Albrecht L, Bourcier M, Ashkenas J, Papp K, Shear N, Toole J, et al. Topical psoriasis therapy in the age of biologics: evidence-based treatment recommendations. J Cutan Med Surg. 2011 Nov-Dec;15(6):309-21.

Chapter 7

Quality of Life in Psoriasis

Delia Colombo and Renata Perego

Additional information is available at the end of the chapter

http://dx.doi.org/10.5772/53998

1. Introduction

Psoriasis has a profound impact on patients' everyday life. The burden of the disease extends beyond physical manifestations and includes significant physical, social and psychological impairment. Numerous studies have demonstrated the significant negative impact of psoriasis on quality of life (QoL) [1-5]. Furthermore, as a chronic disease, psoriasis affects the QoL of both patients and their close relatives in a cumulative way [6]. The family members of patients with psoriasis experience a wide range of detrimental effects on their lives with regards to psychological social and lifestyle modifications, interpersonal relationships, financial issues, family activities, sleep and issues related to the practical care of the patients.

Various factors may contribute to the lower QoL of patients with psoriasis. The chronic nature of the disease and the lack of control over unexpected outbreaks of the symptoms are among the most bothersome aspects of psoriasis [7]. Patients may feel humiliated when they need to expose their bodies during intimate relationships, swimming, using public showers, or anyway living in conditions that do not provide adequate privacy [8]. Thus psoriasis affects patients' social life, daily activities, and sexual functioning [9]. Treatment of psoriasis, as it may be associated with risk for adverse effects, is also an important component of the QoL of psoriasis patients [10]. By utilizing the Short Form-36 (SF-3 6), a generic QoL instrument, it has been demonstrated that psoriasis may cause as much disability as other major medical diseases, including heart disease, diabetes, and cancer [11].

Psoriasis is also related to several co-morbidities, especially cardiovascular diseases and psychiatric disorders. Moreover, cardiovascular risk factors are strongly associated with the severity of inflammation and the duration of disease [12-14].

Improving the QoL in psoriasis patients is an extremely important goal. Therefore, the interventions to improve the process of care of this population should also assess QoL outcomes, such as social functioning and emotional well-being, adjusting for the effects of co-existing chronic conditions. Disease-specific measures may be sensitive enough to detect and quantify small changes that are important to clinicians and patients [15]. Healthcare professionals have a crucial role in identifying and supporting affected patients and families. In order to establish a good relationship with family members and to be able to improve patients' compliance, dermatologists should develop greater insight into the lives of psoriasis patients and their relatives.

In this chapter, the impact of the different aspects of psoriasis on QoL will be reviewed.

2. Skin symptoms

Research found that large percentages of patients with psoriasis reported considerably skin pain and discomfort [16,17]. Skin pain was reported by up to 42%, and skin discomfort by up to 37% of psoriasis patients [16, 18,19]. Skin pain and discomfort had a negative impact on functions such as sleep, mood and enjoyment of life [16]. Studies suggested that other psoriasis-related sensory skin symptoms were associated with sleep disturbances, psychological distress and impaired health related QoL (HRQoL) [20-25].

Ljosaa et al. [17] showed that physiological factors such as skin pain and disease severity were significantly associated with HRQoL and that the association between skin pain and HRQoL was partly mediated by sleep disturbance, while less by psychological distress.

Other skin symptoms of psoriasis can significantly affect physical functioning, perception of disease, and QoL. These symptoms include itching, "skin shedding", tightness, redness, dryness, and bleeding [2, 21]. In particular, a direct correlation between pruritus severity and depression has been shown [26]. Psoriatic lesions of the vulva were found in women with psoriasis, resulting in itching, burning and vulvar discomfort, and women with these symptoms more frequently demonstrated depressive symptoms [27].

Psoriatic skin lesions are often perceived by patients as making their physical appearance unsightly; skin lesions make them feeling disfigured and apprehensive that others will avoid or exclude them, resulting in low self-esteem and self-confidence [28, 29].

When psoriasis involves the palms and soles, which occurs in approximately 40% of patients, the pain and discomfort result in significantly greater physical disability than is experienced by patients without palmoplantar involvement [30]. Nail involvement, which is present in up to 50% of patients, may also limit daily activities such as basic self-care activities and housekeeping [31, 32].

3. Psoriatic arthritis

Psoriatic arthritis (PsA) is a painful disease of the joints and connective tissue affecting 10-30% of patients with psoriasis, and is mainly localized at fingers, toes, wrists, hips and back [2, 3, 31, 33]. PsA can result in damage to bone and synovial membranes, pronounced disability, and increased mortality [33]. Patients with PsA have a significantly worse QoL than those without PsA, as measured by different questionnaires [31, 34].

4. Psychological disturbances and psychiatric co-morbidities

Psoriasis is associated with a variety of psychological difficulties, including poor self-esteem, sexual dysfunction, anxiety, depression, and suicidal ideation [35]. The psychiatric morbidity in psoriasis may be primary or secondary to the impact of the disease upon the patients' QoL.

High depression/anxiety scores, obsessionality and difficulties with verbal expression of emotions, especially anger, social stigmatization, high stress levels, depression, and other psychosocial co-morbidities experienced by patients with psoriasis are not always proportional to, or predicted by, other measurements of disease severity, such as body surface area involvement or plaque severity [36-46]. In general, psychological disturbances, including perception of stigmatization and depression, are stronger determinants of disability in psoriasis patients than are disease severity, location and duration [47]. The Italian PSYCHAE study, which measured psychological distress (PD) in 1580 patients with psoriasis by the General Health Questionnaire-12 (GSQ-12) and the Brief Symptom Inventory (BSI), found that there was no association between disease severity and PD [48].

It is not surprising that perceived stress in patients with psoriasis, as well as with other chronic disease, predicts poorer QoL [49]. On the other hand psoriasis is generally thought to be made worse by stress. Various studies have reported an association between stress and psoriasis. In a study of 132 patients with psoriasis, 39% recalled a significant stressful event within one month before the first episode of psoriasis [50]. In contrast, a more recent prospective clinical study demonstrated that there was no direct relationship between stress and exacerbation of psoriasis, showed no clear relationship between stress levels and worsening of psoriasis and found no time relationships between stress and the appearance of psoriasis [51]. A factor analysis of the Psoriasis Life Stress Inventory revealed two stress-related factors contributing to the psychosocial impact of psoriasis: stress associated with anticipation of the reaction and avoidance by others, and stress associated with patients' experience or beliefs about being evaluated exclusively on the basis of their skin [52]. So, stress is largely secondary to the cosmetic disfigurement associated with psoriasis, with great impact on QoL and possibly resulting in psychological morbidity.

Studies on the relationship between psychological factors and psoriasis severity have primarily been focused on depression, with conflicting results: some authors have found depression correlated with objective measures of disease severity [49], while others have not [53]. Anyway, relatively high rates of depression are reported in patients with psoriasis [54, 55]. Controlled studies found notably higher degree of depression in patients with psoriasis than in controls [56-58].

Suicidal ideation and cases of completed suicide have been reported in psoriasis. The prevalence of suicidal ideation has been reported to be 2.5% among less severely affected outpatients with <30% of their body surface involved and 7.2% among the more severely affected inpatients as compared to 5.2% in acne patients, 2.1% in atopic dermatitis patients and 0% in alopecia areata patients [57, 59]. Death wishes and suicidal ideation were associated with higher depression scores.

Some reports suggest a higher prevalence of alcohol abuse and cigarette smoking among psoriatic patients [60,61]. In one study, there was an 18% prevalence of alcoholism in patients with psoriasis compared to 2% among dermatologic controls [60]. Several studies have shown that treatment outcomes are worse in heavy drinkers [62-64]. Abstinence alone has been shown to possibly induce psoriasis remission, whereas restarting drinking may cause disease relapse [62, 65].

Concerning the evolution of PD in psoriasis, the longitudinal phase of the PSYCHAE study, that specifically evaluated this aspect in 1500 psoriatic patients during up to 12 months, showed that minor PD halved during the observation period, possibly due to improvement of clinical symptoms, while major PD remained stable [66]. The same authors investigated patients' coping strategies and found that planning, active coping and acceptance were strategies most commonly employed by their patients while denial, behavioural disengagement, and substance abuse were the least frequent attitudes [48]. During the 12-month follow-up, active coping and avoiding dramatization by recourse to humor were predictive factors of amelioration of PD [66].

5. Stigma

A stigma is severe social disapproval of a person based on a distinguishing characteristics [67]. It has also been defined as a biologic or social mark that sets a person off from others [68]. Visible lesions cause feelings of stigmatization which can lead to psychological stress and social withdrawal [69]. Psoriasis patients, even those with relatively mild symptoms, experience high stigmatization as compared to sufferers of other skin diseases, with significant impact on outcomes such as QoL, depression and disability [70-72]. Stigmatization has many forms: Ginsburg and Link identified different dimensions, including anticipation of rejection, feeling of being flawed, sensitivity to others' attitude, guilt and shame, reduction of self-esteem [73].

Among the themes at the basis of the stigma experience, shame has an important role. In different studies, patients with psoriasis reported feelings of embarrassment and shame compared to healthy controls [74, 75]. Shame is one of the most reported emotions, especially by women and by patients with a long disease duration [74]. Feelings of shame can have a strong impact on social life, since they can result in avoidance of public spaces, thus reducing social opportunities, even concerning employment [76].

http://dx.doi.org/10.5772/53998

Boehm et al. [67] have found that it is stigmatization that mediates between symptom severity and QoL, in particular the stigmatization parameters 'reduction of self-esteem' and 'rejection'.

6. Gender

Psoriasis does not discriminate by gender. Studies generally show no difference in the severity of physical symptoms suffered by men and women. However, women and men have different subjective perceptions of how symptoms affect their social interactions, emotional states and, ultimately, their QoL.

Men can find it easier to distance themselves from the social effects of psoriasis. Women, in contrast, are more likely to report feeling 'upset', 'disturbed' or 'ashamed' in social settings [77]. Stress research provides another way of understanding differences between men and women's reactions to psoriasis. Women may be more prone to perceive stress and may be more likely to perceive a greater impact on mental QoL [78].Other authors have shown that women may have a higher likelihood of being stress-reactors [79]. Boehm et al. [67] have found that women reported higher discomfort levels and higher stigmatization, and that, in general, gender differences are observable in the mental component summary score, but not in general-physical or skin-related QoL. The PSYCHAE study, conducted on nearly 1600 Italian psoriasis patients, found that the female gender was the most important predictive factor for psychological distress [48].

7. Sexual health

Psoriasis may involve genital skin. In a Netherlands study, of 1943 patients with psoriasis, over 45% reported genital involvement at some time during the course of the disease [80]. Relatively few studies have evaluated the impact of psoriasis on sexual health, however, according to these studies, psoriasis interferes with sexual relations in 35-50% of patients [76, 81, 82]. Sexual dysfunction and distress are particularly high when genital skin is affected.

Psoriasis has a negative influence on a patient's desire for physical intimacy [83] and causes decreased libido in a substantial proportion of patients [81]. Feelings of shame and embarrassment about physical appearance and reduced sexual desire might play a major role in high distress and dysfunction scores in specific sexual indexes [84]. Impairment of sexual activity is more profound in patients with more severe psoriatic symptoms [85], and appears to be more prevalent in women [1]. The patients who believe psoriasis has a negative effect on their sexual lives have more symptoms of depression [81].

Also the treatments used by patients with psoriasis may cause sexual dysfunction: some publications report that antipsoriatic medication such as methotrexate and etretinate might cause sexual impotence and erectile dysfunction [86-88].

8. Impact of QoL on healthcare resources

Psoriasis causes significant occupational disability. Over 17% of patients aged 18-54 report psychologic effects in the workplace due to their disease [2], 6% of employed patients with severe psoriasis reported workplace discrimination [2], and 23% reported that psoriasis affected their choice of career [9]. Problems in work were more frequent in patients with palmoplantar psoriasis. Thus, it appears that psoriasis may have a negative impact on work both for psychological and clinical reasons [2, 9]. Wu et al [89] showed that psoriasis patients were more likely to have missed work for health-related reasons, had significantly more health-related work productivity impairment, and more overall work impairment [90]. This can have financial consequences and may limit lifetime earning potential and career. One study found that 86% of patients with severe psoriasis were 'moderately' or 'a lot' concerned with the time and costs of treating psoriasis [91]. Moreover, psoriasis prevents some patients from obtaining employment altogether [92]. Two studies in the UK found a lower rate of employment in patients with severe psoriasis [41, 92]. Patients with psoriasis who are working, however, tend to have a low work QoL [91]. Fleischer et al [93] theorized that the effect of psoriasis on a patient's work life might result in reduced socio-economical standing and limitations and 34% of the study patients reported hardships due to the financial burden of the disease.

9. Impact of QoL on healthcare resources

Poorer QoL of psoriasis patients is associated with increased healthcare resource utilization, independent of the clinical severity of the disease [94]. As stated previously in this chapter, measuring clinical severity of skin lesions does not fully capture the effect of the disease on patient QoL [47, 95].

The study by Sato et al. [94] showed that healthcare resource utilization by European patients with plaque psoriasis, in terms of dermatologist visits and hospitalizations, is greater for those with poorer QoL, independent of clinical disease severity, and may decrease if QoL improves. These authors also found that poor QoL is also associated with employment disadvantages, even when controlling for disease severity, suggesting that indirect costs of psoriasis may also be augmented for patients who have a poor QoL.

10. QoL in children with psoriasis

In childhood, QoL is greatly influenced by psoriasis. Data on QoL in juvenile psoriasis are limited, however some studies demonstrated the negative influence of psoriasis on the QoL of children by means of the Children's Dermatology Life Quality Index (CDLQI) [96-100].The social development domain, which is one of the developmental milestones in a child, is particularly impaired [101]. Moreover, psoriasis in childhood causes a high degree of limitations on recreational activities in at least 15-30% of patients [101]. Itching and problems with treatments were shown to have the highest impact on the children's QoL. The same authors showed that QoL in the long term is not determined by the age of onset of psoriasis.

Other authors demonstrated that the significant negative impact of plaque psoriasis on QoL of children with psoriasis is generally comparable to the impact of other serious pediatric chronic diseases, as arthritis, asthma, and diabetes [102]. The impairment in QoL impacts particularly emotional and school functioning [102].

11. Impact of psoriasis treatments on QoL

Only a few clinical trials have been conducted on the effect of treatments for psoriasis on QoL and some of them were not specifically designed to measure QoL but rather inferred the drug impact on QoL from its effect on the clinical symptoms of the disease.

Among topical treatments, calcipotriol-betamethasone gel was reported to improve QoL in patients with scalp psoriasis [103]. Narrowband ultraviolet B (NBUVB) phototherapy administered three times a week for 6 months significantly improved QoL in 95 plaque-type psoriasis patients [104].

Low-dose (3 mg/kg/day), short-term cyclosporine therapy was effective in improving QoL as measured by Skindex-16 and GHQ-28 in 41 patients with mild to severe psoriasis [105]. An Italian longitudinal study on psoriasis patients followed up for 12 months observed that treatment with cyclosporine significantly reduced by 30% the risk for minor psychological distress, while methotrexate and topical corticosteroids were associated with significantly increased risks (33% and 185%, respectively) [66]. Additionally, results from a small study indicate that the use of cyclosporine for the treatment of nail psoriasis can lead to an improvement in QoL [106].

In a Canadian randomized, placebo-controlled trial on 451 plaque psoriasis patients, voclosporin was reported to improve QoL, assessed by DLQI and Psoriasis Disability Index (PDI) [107].

A recent analysis of Japanese trials on infliximab demonstrates that a Psoriasis Area and Severity Index (PASI) 90 response is necessary to achieve a DLQI of 0 or 1. Since infliximab showed to achieve nearly 50% of PASI 90 responses, the authors infer that it might be useful in meeting the goal of a DLQI of 0 or 1 [108].

An analysis of pooled data from two randomized, placebo-controlled trials evaluated the effects of adalimumab on the risk of symptom worsening in psoriasis and the subsequent impact on HRQoL. The analysis pointed out that clinically relevant worsening of psoriasis symptoms was associated with substantial worsening of HRQoL. Adalimumab treatment was associated with a reduction in risk of clinical worsening of psoriasis, but its specific effect on HRQoL was not reported [109].

A metanalysis of randomized, controlled trials of etanercept in patients with rheumatoid arthritis, psoriatic arthritis and psoriasis, evaluating among other outcome measures the effect of the drug on HRQoL, treatment with etanercept resulted in improvements in the physical and mental component summary scores (PCS and MCS), as well as in individual SF-36 domains across all indications [110]. The PRESTA trial, conducted in Germany, evaluated the effect of etanercept on a composite measure of skin symptoms, joint manifestations, and QoL [111]. At 24 weeks, around 30% of patients met the triad of efficacy outcomes. In juvenile plaque psoriasis, one randomized, controlled, longitudinal study described a significant positive effect of etanercept on QoL [100].

In a subanalysis of the PHOENIX 1 and 2 trials on ustekinumab in psoriasis, aimed at evaluating the effect on HRQoL and sexual difficulties, ustekinumab treatment was associated with significant improvement in HRQoL and sexual difficulties due to psoriasis [112]. Another post-hoc analysis of the PHOENIX 2 trial showed that ustekinumab decreases work limitations, improves work productivity and reduces work days missed in the 1230 study patients with moderate-to-severe psoriasis [113]. The efficacy of ustekinumab was also evaluated in nail psoriasis and nail-associated QoL in a population treated for cutaneous psoriasis. Together with a statistically significant reduction of the nail psoriasis severity index (NAPSI), a significant improvement of the international onychomycosis QoL scores was observed at all time points up to 40 weeks [114].

In children, in a psoriatic cohort treated in daily clinical practice, QoL was assessed by CDLQI. The results showed that all psoriasis treatments contributed to a significant improvement in children's QoL, which was greatest with dithranol and systemic treatments. The highest positive impact with all treatments was observed on itching and sleep disturbances [115].

12. Conclusions and recommendations for clinical practice

Psoriasis is associated with significant psychological distress, psychiatric morbidity, experience of stigmatization and decreased QoL. Several studies have demonstrated the significant negative impact of psoriasis on QoL, which is similar to the impact of other major chronic diseases as heart diseases, diabetes and cancer. Presence of psoriatic arthritis, psychiatric disorders, and other co-morbidities may further worsen QoL and should be taken into account. The association between symptom severity and QoL, though observed by some studies [98,116], is not always strong, and other studies found no significant association at all [48, 95]. Symptom severity has been shown to have a greater direct impact on the physical rather than the mental components of QoL, while the effects of stigmatization on QoL are more strongly mental [67]. Some research has concluded that 'subjective experience of psoriasis is a more powerful determinant of QoL' in comparison to clinical measures [117].

Studies have shown that dermatologists employ a problem-orientated coping style in caring' for their patients, and often appear much more interested in investigating the superficial skin rather than the deep emotions of their patients [48]. On the contrary, it is essential that measures of psychosocial morbidity are included when assessing psoriasis severity.

In clinical practice there is a great challenge for dermatologists to improve the QoL of adults and children with psoriasis. Greater attention should be paid to the possible limitations that these patients experience. The outcome of QoL measurements should be taken into account when deciding on treatment strategies. Dermatology professionals should be encouraged to identify patients, irrespective of gender and of severity of clinical manifestations, who perceive especially high levels of discomfort, indicate problems in maintaining self-esteem and/or have experienced instances of rejection. Specific therapeutic strategies that address issues of self-esteem and social rejection are appropriate especially for these patients. Optimal therapy that leads to long-lasting remission can only be achieved by addressing both the physical and psychosocial effects of psoriasis. The choice of the optimal psoriasis treatment should also take into account the effect of the drug on the patient's psychosocial well-being, and adjunctive psychological interventions before and during treatment may be of benefit for selected patients. It is recommended that psoriasis patients, especially those with severe disease, receive a more holistic, multitarget approach that encompasses both medical and psychological measures.

Author details

Delia Colombo and Renata Perego

Luigi Marchesi Hospital, Inzago - Milan, Italy

References

[1] De Arruda LH, De Moares AP. The impact of psoriasis on quality of life. Br J Dermatol 2001; 144:33–6

[2] Krueger G, Koo J, Lebwohl M et al. The impact of psoriasis on quality of life: results of a 1998 National Psoriasis Foundation patient-membership survey. Arch Dermatol 2001; 137:280–4

[3] Zachariae R, Zachariae H, Blomqvist K et al. Quality of life in 6497 Nordic patients with psoriasis. Br J Dermatol 2002; 146:1006–16

[4] Mease PJ, Menter MA. Quality-of-life issues in psoriasis and psoriatic arthritis: outcome measures and therapies from a dermatological perspective. J Am Acad Dermatol 2006; 54: 685–704.

[5] Mukhtar R, Choi J, Koo JY. Quality-of-life issues in psoriasis. Dermatol Clin 2004; 22: 389–395.

[6] Tadros A, Vergou T, Stratigos A et al. Psoriasis: is it the tip of the iceberg for the quality of life of patients and their families? Eur Acad Dermatol Venereol 2011; 25:1282–7

[7] Gelfand JM, Feldman SR, Stern RS et al. Determinants of quality of life in patients with psoriasis: a study from the US population. J Am Acad Dermatol 2004; 51:704–8

[8] Fortune DG, Richards HL, Griffiths CE. Psychologic factors in psoriasis: consequences, mechanisms, and interventions. Dermatol Clin 2005; 23:681–94

[9] Weiss SC, Kimball AB, Liewehr DJ et al. Quantifying the harmful effect of psoriasis on health-related quality of life. J Am Acad Dermatol 2002; 47:512–8

[10] Feldman SR, Koo JY, Menter A et al. Decision points for the initiation of systemic treatment for psoriasis. J Am Acad Dermatol 2005; 53:101–7

[11] Rapp SR, Feldman SR, Exum ML et al. Psoriasis causes as much disability as other major medical diseases. J Am Acad Dermatol 1999; 41:401–7

[12] Kimball AB, Guerin A, Mulani P et al. The risk of coronary heart disease and stroke among psoriasis patients. Abstract P 3369 AAD. J Am Acad Dermatol 2009; 60: Suppl AB179.

[13] Ludwig RJ, Herzog C, Rostock A et al. Psoriasis: a possible risk factor for development of coronary artery calcification. Br J Dermatol 2007; 156: 271–276.

[14] Neimann AL, Shin DB, Wang X, Margolis DJ, Troxel AB, Gelfand JM. Prevalence of cardiovascular risk factors in patients with psoriasis. J Am Acad Dermatol 2006; 55: 829–835.

[15] Patrick DL, Deyo RA. Generic and disease-specific measures in assessing health status and quality of life. Med Care 1989; 27[3 Suppl):S217–32

[16] Ljosaa TM, Rustoen T, Mork C et al. Skin pain and discomfort in psoriasis: an exploratory study of symptom prevalence and characteristics. Acta Derm Venereol 2010; 90: 39–45.

[17] Ljosaa TM, Mork C, Stubhaug A, Mourn T, Wahl AK. Skin pain and skin discomfort is associated with quality of life in patients with psoriasis. J Eur Acad Dermatol Venereol 2012; 26:29-35

[18] Sampogna F, Gisondi P, Melchi CF, Amerio P, Girolomoni G, Abeni D. Prevalence of symptoms experienced by patients with different clinical types of psoriasis. Br J Dermatol 2004; 151: 594–599.

[19] McKenna KE, Stern RS. The impact of psoriasis on the quality of life of patients from the 16-center PUVA follow-up cohort. J Am Acad Dermatol 1997; 36: 388–394.

[20] Fortune DG, Richards HL, Griffiths CE. Psychologic factors in psoriasis: consequences, mechanisms, and interventions. Dermatol Clin 2005; 23: 681–694.

[21] Yosipovitch G, Goon A, Wee J, Chan YH, Goh CL. The prevalence and clinical characteristics of pruritus among patients with extensive psoriasis. Br J Dermatol 2000; 143: 969–973.

[22] Globe D, Bayliss MS, Harrison DJ. The impact of itch symptoms in psoriasis: results from physician interviews and patient focus groups. Health Qual Life Outcomes 2009; 7: 62.

[23] Choi J, Koo JY. Quality of life issues in psoriasis. J Am Acad Dermatol 2003; 49: 57–61.

[24] Zachariae R, Zachariae C, Ibsen HH, Mortensen JT, Wulf HC. Psychological symptoms and quality of life of dermatology outpatients and hospitalized dermatology patients. Acta Derm Venereol 2004; 84: 205–212.

[25] Wahl A, Moum T, Hanestad BR, Wiklund I. The relationship between demographic and clinical variables and quality of life aspects in patients with psoriasis. Qual Life Res 1999; 8: 319–326.

[26] Gupta MA, Gupta AK, Schork NJ, Ellis CN. Depression modulates pruritus perception: a study of pruritus in psoriasis, atopic dermatitis, and chronic idiopathic urticaria. Psychosom Med 1994; 56: 36–40.

[27] Zamirska A, Reich A, Berny-Moreno J, et al. Vulvar pruritus and burning sensation in women with psoriasis. Acta Derm Venereol 2008; 88: 132–135.

[28] McHenry PM, Doherty VR. Psoriasis: an audit of patients' views on the disease and its treatment. Br J Dermatol 1992; 127: 13–17.

[29] Koo J. Population-based epidemiologic study of psoriasis with emphasis on quality of life assessment. Dermatol Clin 1996; 14: 485–496.

[30] Pettey AA, Balkrishnan R, Rapp SR, et al. Patients with palmoplantar psoriasis have more physical disability and discomfort than patients with other forms of psoriasis: implications for clinical practice. J Am Acad Dermatol 2003; 49: 271–275.

[31] National Psoriasis Foundation Data. 2004; [online]. Available at: http://www.psoriasis.org/.

[32] de Jong EM, Seegers BA, Gulinck MK, et al. Psoriasis of the nails associated with disability in a large number of patients: results of a recent interview with 1728 patients. Dermatology 1996; 193: 300–303.

[33] Gladman DD, Rahman P. Psoriatic arthritis. In: Ruddy S, Harris ED, Sledge CB, et al., eds. Kelley's Textbook of Rheumatology, 6th edn. Philadelphia, PA: WB Saunders Company, 2001: 1071–1078.

[34] Rosen CF, Mussani F, Chandran V, Eder L, Thavaneswaran A, Gladman DD. Patients with psoriatic arthritis have worse quality of life than those with psoriasis alone. Rheumatology (Oxford) 2012; 51:571-6

[35] Basavaraj , Navya MA, Rashmi R. Stress and quality of life in psoriasis: an update. Int J Dermatol 2011; 50:783-92.

[36] Gupta MA, Gupta AK, Watteel GN. Early onset (<age 40 years) psoriasis is associated with greater psychopathology than late onset psoriasis. Acta Derm Venereol 1996; 76: 464–466.

[37] Niemeier V, Nippesen M, Kupfer J, et al. Psychological factors associated with hand dermatoses: which subgroup needs additional psychological care? Br J Dermatol 2002; 146: 1031–1037.

[38] Skevington SM, Bradshaw J, Hepplewhite A, et al. How does psoriasis affect quality of life? Assessing an Ingram-regimen outpatient programme and validating the WHOQOL-100. Br J Dermatol 2006; 154: 680–691.

[39] Feldman SR, Fleischer AB Jr, Reboussin DM, et al. The economic impact of psoriasis increases with psoriasis severity. J Am Acad Dermatol 1997; 37: 564–569.

[40] Kirkby B, Richards HL, Woo P, et al. Physical and psychological measures are necessary to assess overall psoriasis severity. J Am Acad Dermatol 2001; 45:72–76.

[41] Fortune DG, Main CJ, O'Sullivan TM, Griffiths CE. Quality of life in patients with psoriasis: the contribution of clinical variables and psoriasis-specific stress. Br J Dermatol 1997; 137: 755–760.

[42] Gupta MA, Gupta AK, Haberman HF. Psoriasis and psychiatry: an update. Gen Hosp Psychiatry 1987; 9:157–166.

[43] Matussek P, Agerer D, Seibt G. Aggression in depressives and psoriatics. Psychother Psychosom 1985;43: 120–125.

[44] Rubino IA, Sonnino A, Pezzarossa B, et al. Personality disorders and psychiatric symptoms in psoriasis. Psychol Rep 1995; 77: 547–553.

[45] Vidoni D, Campiutti E, D'Aronco R, et al. Psoriasis and alexithymia. Acta Derm Venereol (Stockh) 1989; 146:91–92.

[46] Kimball AB, Jacobson C, Weiss S, et al. The psychosocial burden of psoriasis. Am J Clin Dermatol 2005; 6: 383–392.

[47] Richards HL, Fortune DG, Griffiths CE, Main CJ. The contribution of perceptions of stigmatisation to disability in patients with psoriasis. J Psychosom Res 2001; 50:11–15.

[48] Finzi A, Colombo D, Caputo A, Andreassi L, Chimenti S, Vena G, Simoni L, Sgarbi S, Giannetti A for the PSYCHAE Study Group.Psychological distress and coping strategies in patients with psoriasis: the PSYCHAE Study. J Eur Acad Dermatol Venereol 2007; 21:1161-9

[49] O'Leary CJ, Creamer D, Higgins E, Weinman J. Perceived stress, stress attributions and psychological distress in psoriasis. J Psychosom Res 2004; 57: 465–471.

[50] Polenghi MM, Molinari E, Gala C, et al. Experience with psoriasis in a psychosomatic dermatology clinic.Acta Derm Venereol (Stockh) 1994; 186: 65–66.

[51] Berg M, Svensson M, Brandberg M, Nordlind K. Psoriasis and stress: a prospective study. J Eur Acad Dermatol Venereol 2008; 22: 670–674.

[52] Fortune DG, Main CJ, O'Sullivan TM, Griffiths CE. Assessing illness-related stress in psoriasis: the psychometric properties of the Psoriasis Life Stress Inventory. J Psychosom Res 1997; 42: 467–475.

[53] Schmitt JM, Ford DE. Role of depression in quality of life for patients with psoriasis. Dermatology 2007; 215:17-27

[54] Bouguéon K, Misery L. Depression and psoriasis. Ann Dermatol Venereol 2008; 135: 254–258.

[55] Van Voorhees AS, Fried R. Depression and quality of life in psoriasis. Postgrad Med 2009; 121: 154–161

[56] Hardy GE, Cotterill JA. A study of depression and obsessionality in dysmorphophobic and psoriasis patients. Br J Psychiatry 1982; 140: 19–22.

[57] Gupta MA, Gupta AK Depression and suicidal ideation in dermatology patients with acne, alopecia areata, atopic dermatitis and psoriasis. Br J Dermatol 1998; 139: 846–850.

[58] Devrimci-Ozguven H, Kundakci TN, Kumbasar H, Boyvat A. The depression, anxiety, life satisfaction and affective expression levels in psoriasis patients. J Eur Acad Dermatol Venereol 2000; 14: 267–271.

[59] Gupta MA, Schork NJ, Gupta AK, et al. Suicidal ideation in psoriasis. Int J Dermatol 1993; 32: 188–190.

[60] Morse RM, Perry HO, Hurt RD. Alcoholism and psoriasis. Alcohol Clin Exp Res 1985; 9: 396–399.

[61] Mills CM, Srivastava RD, Harvey IM, et al. Smoking habits in psoriasis: a case control study. Br J Dermatol 1992; 127: 18–21.

[62] Higgins EM, du Vivier AW. Alcohol abuse and treatment resistance in skin disease [letter]. J Am Acad Dermatol 1994; 30: 1048.

[63] Higgins EM, du Vivier AW. Cutaneous disease and alcohol misuse. Br Med Bull 1994; 50: 85–98.

[64] Gupta MA, Schork NJ, Gupta AK, Ellis CN. Alcohol intake and treatment responsiveness of psoriasis: a prospective study. J Am Acad Dermatol 1993; 28:730–732.

[65] Vincenti GE, Blunden SM. Psoriasis and alcohol abuse. J R Army Med Corps 1987; 133: 77–78.

[66] Colombo D, Caputo A, Finzi A et al for the PSYCHAE Study Group. Evolution of and risk factors for psychological distress in patients with psoriasis: the PSYCHAE study. Int J Immunopathol Pharmacol 2010; 23:297-306

[67] Boehm D, Stock Gissendanner S, Bangemann K et al. Perceived relationships between severity of psoriasis symptoms, gender, stigmatization and quality of life. J Eur Acad Dermatol Venereol 2012; DOI: 10.1111/j.1468-3083.2012.04451.x

[68] Jones E, Farina A, Hastorf A, Markus H, Miller D. Social stigma: the psychology of marked relationships. New York: Freeman, 1984

[69] Hrehorow E, Salomon J, Matusiak L et al. Patients with psoriasis feel stigmatized. Acta Derm Venereol 2011; 92: 67–72.

[70] Gupta MA, Gupta AK, Watteel GN. Perceived deprivation of social touch in psoriasis is associated with greater psychologic morbidity: an index of the stigma experience in dermatologic disorders. Cutis 1998; 61:339–342.

[71] Richards HL, Fortune DG, Griffiths CE, Main CJ. The contribution of perceptions of stigmatisation to disability in patients with psoriasis 26. J Psychosom Res 2001; 50:11–15.

[72] Schmid-Ott G, Jaeger B, Kuensebeck HW et al. Dimensions of stigmatization in patients with psoriasis in a 'Questionnaire on Experience with Skin Complaints' 31. Dermatology 1996; 193: 304–310.

[73] Ginsburg IH, Link BG. Feelings of stigmatization in patients with psoriasis. J Am Acad Dermatol 1989; 20: 53–63.

[74] Sampogna F, Tabolli S, Abeni D, and the IDI Multipurpose Psoriasis Research on Vital Experiences (IMPROVE) Investigators. Living with psoriasis: prevalence of shame, anger, worry, and problems in daily activities and social life. Acta Derm Venereol 2012; 92:299-303

[75] Magin P, Adams J, Heading G, Pond D, Smith W. The psychological sequelae of psoriasis: results of a qualitative study. Psychol Health Med 2009; 14:150-61

[76] Weiss SC, Kimball AB, Liewehr DJ, Blauwelt A, Turner ML, Emanuel EJ. Quantifying the harmful effect of psoriasis on health-related quality of life. J Am Acad Dermatol 2002; 47:512-8

[77] Perrott SB, Murray AH, Lowe J, Ruggiero KM. The personal-group discrimination discrepancy in persons living with psoriasis. Basic Appl Social Psychol 2000; 22: 57–67.

[78] Misery L, Thomas L, Jullien D et al. Comparative study of stress and quality of life in outpatients consulting for different dermatoses in 5 academic departments of dermatology. Eur J Dermatol 2008; 18: 412–415.

[79] Zachariae R, Zachariae H, Blomqvist K et al. Self-reported stress reactivity and psoriasis-related stress of Nordic psoriasis sufferers. J Eur Acad Dermatol Venereol 2004; 18: 27–36.

[80] Meeuwis KA, de Hullu JA, de Jager ME et al. Genital psoriasis: a questionnaire-based survey on a concealed skin disease in the Netherlands. J Eur Acad Dermatol Venereol 2010; 24:1425–30.

[81] Gupta MA, Gupta AK. Psoriasis and sex: a study of moderately to severely affected patients. Int J Dermatol 1997; 36: 259–262.

[82] Ramsay B, O'Reagan M. A survey of the social and psychological effects of psoriasis. Br J Dermatol 1988; 118: 195–201.

[83] Wahl AK, Gjengedal E, Hanestad BR. The bodily suffering of living with severe psoriasis: in-depth interviews with 22 hospitalized patients with psoriasis. Qual Health Res 2002; 12: 250–261.

[84] Meeuwis KA, de Hullu JA, van de Nieuwenhof HP, Evers AW, Massuger LF, van de Kerkhof PC, van Rossum MM. Quality of life and sexual health in patients with genital psoriasis. Br J Dermatol 2011; 164: 1247-55

[85] Koo J. Population-based epidemiologic study of psoriasis with emphasis on quality of life assessment. Dermatol Clin 1996; 14:483-96

[86] Aguirre MA, Velez A, Romero M et al. Gynecomastia and sexual impotence associated with methotrexate treatment. J Rheumatol 2002; 29:1793–4.

[87] Reynolds OD. Erectile dysfunction in etretinate treatment. Arch Dermatol 1991; 127:425–6.

[88] Wylie G, Evans CD, Gupta G. Reduced libido and erectile dysfunction: rarely reported side-effects of methotrexate. Clin Exp Dermatol 2009; 34:e234.

[89] Wu Y, Mills D, Bala M. Impact of psoriasis on patients' work and productivity: a retrospective, matched case-control analysis. Am J Clin Dermatol 2009; 10:407-10

[90] Horn EJ, Fox KM, Patel V, chiou CF, Dann F, Lebwohl M. Association of patient-reported psoriasis severity with income and employment. J Am Acad Dermatol 2007; 57:963-71

[91] Feldman SR, Fleischer AB Jr, Reboussin DM, et al. The economic impact of psoriasis increases with psoriasis severity. J Am Acad Dermatol 1997; 37:564–569.

[92] Finlay AY, Coles EC. The effect of severe psoriasis on the quality of life of 369 patients. Br J Dermatol 1995; 132: 236–244.

[93] Fleischer AB Jr, Feldman SR, Bradham DD. Office-based physician services provided by dermatologists in the United States in 1990. J Invest Dermatol 1994; 102:93–97.

[94] Sato R, Milligan G, Molta C, Singh A. Health-related quality of life and healthcare resource use in European patients with plaque psoriasis: an association independent of observed disease severity. Clin Exper Dermatol 2010; 36:24-28

[95] Perrott SB, Murray AH, Lowe J, Mathieson CM. The psychosocial impact of psoriasis: physical severity, quality of life, and stigmatization. Physiol Behav 2000; 70: 567–71.

[96] Lewis-Jones MS, Finlay AY. The Children's Dermatology Life Quality Index (CDLQI): initial validation and practical use. Br J Dermatol 1995; 132:942–9.

[97] Beattie PE, Lewis-Jones MS. A comparative study of impairment of quality of life in children with skin disease and children with other chronic childhood diseases. Br J Dermatol 2006; 155:145–51.

[98] de Jager ME, van de Kerkhof PC, de Jong EM et al. A cross-sectional study using the Children's Dermatology Life Quality Index (CDLQI) in childhood psoriasis: negative effect on quality of life and moderate correlation of CDLQI with severity scores. Br J Dermatol 2010; 163:1099–101.

[99] Ganemo A, Wahlgren CF, Svensson A. Quality of life and clinical features in Swedish children with psoriasis. Pediatr Dermatol 2011; 28:375–9.

[100] Langley RG, Paller AS, Hebert AA et al. Patient-reported outcomes in pediatric patients with psoriasis undergoing etanercept treatment: 12-week results from a phase III randomized controlled trial. J Am Acad Dermatol 2011; 64:64–70.

[101] De Jager ME, de Jong EM, van de Kerkhof PC, Evers AE, Seyger MM. An intrapatient comparison of quality of life in psoriasis in childhood and adulthood. J Eur Acad Dermatol Venereol 2011; 25:828-31

[102] Varni JW, Globe DR, Gandra SR, Harrison DJ, Hooper M, Baumgartner S. Health-related quality of life of pediatric patients with moderate to severe plaque psoriasis: comparisons to four common chronic diseases. Eur J Pediatr 2012; 171:485-92

[103] Mrowietz U, Macheleidt O, Eicke C. Effective treatment and improvement of quality of life in patients with scalp psoriasis by topical use of calcipotriol/betamethasone (Xamiol®-gel): results. J Dtsch Dermatol Ges 2011; 9:825-31

[104] Al Robaee AA, Alzolibani AA. Narrowband ultraviolet B phototherapy improves the quality of life in patients with psoriasis. Saudi Med J 2011; 32:603-6

[105] Okubo Y, Natsume S, Usui K, Amaya M, Tsuboi R. Low-dose, short-term ciclosporin (Neoral®) therapy is effective in improving patients' quality of life as assessed by Skindex-16 and GHQ-28 in mild to severe psoriasis patients. J Dermatol 2011;38:465-72

[106] Abe M, Syuto T, Yokoyama Y, Ishikawa O. Improvement of quality of life and clinical usefulness of cyclosporin administration in patients with nail psoriasis. J Dermatol 2011; 38:916-49

[107] Kunynetz R, Carey W, Thomas R, Toth D, Trafford T, vender R. Quality of life in plaque psoriasis patients treated with voclosporin: a Canadian phase III, randomized, multicenter, double-blind, placebo-controlled study. Eur J Dermatol 2011; 21:89-94

[108] Torii H, Sato N, Yoshinari T, Nakagawa H. Dramatic impact of a Psoriasis Area and Severity Index 90 response on the quality of life in patients with psoriasis: an analysis of Japanese clinical trials of infliximab. J Dermatol 2012; 39:253-9

[109] Papp KA, Signorovitch J, Ramakrishnan K, Yu AP, Gupta SR, Bao Y, Mulani PM. Effects of adalimumab versus placebo on risk of symptom worsening in psoriasis and subsequent impacts on health-related quality of life: analysis of pooled data from two randomized, double-blind, placebo –controlled, multicentre clinical trials. Clin Drug Investig 2011; 31:51-60

[110] Strand V, Sharp V, Koenig AS, Park G, Shi Y, Wang B, Zack DJ, Fiorentino D. Comparison of health-related quality of life in rheumatoid arthritis, psoriatic arthritis an psoriasis and effects of etanercept treatment. Ann Rheum Dis 2012; 71:1143-50

[111] Prinz JC, Fitzgerald O, Boggs RI, Foehl J, Robertson D, Pedersen R, Molta CT, Freundlich B. Combination of skin, joint and quality of life outcomes with etanercept in psoriasis and psoriatic arthritis in the PRESTA trial. J Eur Acad Dermatol Venereol 2011; 25:559-64

[112] Guenther L, Han C, Szapary P, Schenkel B, Poulin Y, Bourcier M, Ortonne JP, Sofen HL. Impact of ustekinumab on health-related quality of life and sexual difficulties associated with psoriasis: results from two phase III clinical trials. J Eur Acad Dermatol Venereol 2011; 25:851-7

[113] Reich K, Schenkel B, Zhao N, Szapary P, Augustin M, Bourcier M, Guenther L, Langley RG. Ustekinumab decreases work limitations, improves work productivity, and reduces work days missed in patients with moderate-to-severe psoriasis: results from PHOENIX 2. J Dermatolog Treat 2011; 22:337-47

[114] Rigopoulos D, Gregoriou S, Makris M, Ioannides D. Efficacy of ustekinumab in nail psoriasis and improvement in nail-associated quality of life in a population treated with ustekinumab for cutaneous psoriasis: an open prospective unblended study. Dermatology 2011; 223:325-9

[115] Oostven AM, de Jager ME, ven de Kerkhof PC, Donders AR; de Jong EM, Seyger MM. The influence of treatments in daily clinical practice on the Children's Dermatology Life Quality Index in juvenile psoriasis: a longitudinal study from the Child-CAPTURE patient registry. Br J Dermatol 2012; 167:145-9

[116] Augustin M, Kruger K, Radtke MA et al. Disease severity, quality of life and health care in plaque-type psoriasis: a multicenter cross-sectional study in Germany. Dermatology 2008; 216: 366–372.

[117] Russo PA, Ilchef R, Cooper AJ. Psychiatric morbidity in psoriasis: a review. Australas J Dermatol 2004; 45: 155–159

Chapter 8

Effects of Tonsillectomy on Psoriasis and Tonsil Histology-Ultrastructure

Sebastiano Bucolo, Valerio Torre,
Giuseppe Romano, Carmelo Quattrocchi,
Filippo Farri, Maura Filidoro and Claudio Caldarelli

Additional information is available at the end of the chapter

http://dx.doi.org/10.5772/55978

1. Introduction

Psoriasis is a chronic inflammatory disorder involving both cutaneous and mucous surfaces. Microscopic findings include a reactive abnormal epidermal differentiation, parakeratosis and elongation of rete ridges along with a characteristic mononuclear and neutrophilic inflammatory infiltrate.

Although several clinical variants of psoriasis are well recognized (i.e. guttate psoriasis, pustular psoriasis), the so-called plaque type is the most common type. It mainly affects the extensor limbs surface and the scalp with circular or oval red plaques variable in extention and duration.

Numerous studies indicate subclinical or recurrent streptococcal infection as a trigger or maintenance factor in the pathogenesis of psoriasis in children but although it is well known that guttate psoriasis may be precipitated by streptococcal infection, there is no firm evidence to support the use of antibiotics either in the management of established guttate psoriasis or in preventing its development following streptococcal sore throat. Although both antibiotics and tonsillectomy have frequently been advocated for patients with recurrent guttate Psoriasis or chronic plaque Psoriasis, there is to date no evidence that either intervention is beneficial. Few histological and no ultrastructural studies to date have directly investigated psoriatic effects on palatine tonsils.

The pathophysiology and etiology of psoriasis rest on different and poorly defined mechanisms and conditions mainly related to environmental and genetic factors, the latter related to disease susceptibility. Moreover, additional studies focused on the role of infections as well as bacterial products, toxic or antigenic substances that may act as stimulating factors for polymorphonuclear leukocyte chemotaxis, cytokines and proteolytic enzyme production and T cell response.

The current pilot study attempt to investigate the role of infections in patients with psoriasis and chronic tonsillitis, evaluating the differences among those patients and a non psoriatic control group suffering from chronic tonsillitis, both groups having evidence of beta-haemolytic streptococcal colonization. Clinical data and histological/ultrastructural findings as well as literature data pertaining such a subject were taken into account.

Preliminary date are reported and discussed.

2. Background on tonsil immunology

The tonsil surface is usually covered by stratified squamous epithelium that envelops tonsils to form the crypts. There are generally some 20-30 crypts for tonsil. Within the crypt epithelium is not tightly arranged and presents macrophages, dendritic cells and lymphocytes to epithelial cells interspersed. Furthermore the wall contains cryptic cells micropores (M), which are tubulovescicular in nature and facilitate the internalization of the antigen. Under the epithelium it extends the interfollicular zone, rich in T cells. Moreover this is an area of antigen presentation by interdigitating cells, macrophages, and follicular dendritic cells. The germinal centers of lymphoid follicles are the locations of differentiation and proliferation of B cells.

Immune function itself begins with the effective internalization of the antigen from the pharynx to the tonsillar lymphoid tissue. After the antigen is placed inside a tonsil is processed and presented to T and B lymphocytes. The resulting interaction leads to terminal differentiation of B cells into antibody forming cells and the creation of T and B memory cells. The appropriate sensitization is required for effective immune function and there are multiple systems and many molecules that can induce functions of T and B cells in various extensions. This system works in concert, but, and it is important, the inappropriate reporting can lead to down-regulation of the immune responsiveness of T and B cells. It's therefore necessary to consider the different factors that can lead to modulation of the immune response.

The antigen is internalized in extra follicular areas of the tonsil passing through the M cells localized at the base of the tonsillar crypt. These tubulovescicular cells carry antigens in the tonsil [1]. Dendritic cells and macrophages are also found in the epithelium of cryptic wall. As the M cells they internalize the antigen; however they are also involved in antigen presentation to T cells in the extra follicular areas and the follicles of B cells [2].

Antigen presentation is a complex interaction between the antigen presenting cells and T and B lymphocytes. The first process the antigen and present it bound to the antibody in such a way as to interact with specific molecules on the cell surface of the lymphocytes. The principal antigen presenting cells are macrophages, interdigitating cells and follicular dendritic cells. The macrophages are present both in the epithelium of the crypts and in the germinal centers, as noted with the use of monoclonal antibodies (mAb) MAC 387 and CD68. MAC 387-positive cells were observed in the epithelium of the crypts, while CD68 in extrafollicular areas and germinal centers. These two types of macrophages represent a means for the signaling of B and T cells [3].

The exact nature of the macrophage-lymphocyte signal is not fully known; however it seems to involve a direct cell to cell contact in which the macrophage extends a cytoplasmic process that surrounds the lymphocyte. This interaction depends from the expression by the macrophage antigen MHC class II, which are expressed after activation by the interferon-γ. In addition to interaction with B and T cells, macrophages also interact with follicular dendritic cells through direct contact. Despite the foregoing discussion indicates that macrophages play an important role in antigen presentation, their role in the activation of lymphocytes has not been fully determined. Another antigen presenting cell, the interdigitating cell, that contains S-100 protein, is found more frequently in extrafollicular areas but was found in cryptic epithelium.

Unlike macrophages, it expresses the antigens MCH II without priming by interferon-γ. Such as macrophages, it is found in close contact with helper T cells and it is believed to present the antigen to in maturation T cells. The follicular dendritic cells, which contain the active C3b found on immune complexes, are present in germinal centers and in mantle zones. In these areas, the follicular dendritic cells distribute antigens to B cells, which in turn in germinal centers present the immunogen to T cells. The interaction of the follicular dendritic cell with the B cell can lead to the development of the B cell or a B cell memory, or in a cell secreting immunoglobulins [4].

Along with these antigen-presenting cells, other cells may play a supporting role in the activation of lymphocytes. The cells of the fibroblastic latex, for example, are found in the T cell areas and form a dendritic network [5]. The function of these cells is unknown; however fibroblasts treated with interferon-γ have shown to express antigens of the major histocompatibility complex on their surface. With other signals fibroblasts can play a role in increasing the T cell response to antigenic stimulation.

The successful activation of T and B lymphocytes is the result of complex interactions between 1) the antigen presenting cells and lymphocytes, 2) the accessory cells and lymphocytes, and 3) the T and B lymphocytes. These interactions occur by direct contact or via cytokines. The direct interaction between antigen presenting cells and T cells involves multiple connections[5]. There are numerous determinants of T cells and their respective ligands of antigen presenting cells in tonsil tissues. A main surface molecule of lymphocyte is the determinant C3, structurally related to the T cell receptor (TCR) and subjected to tyrosine phosphorylation of one of its chains upon interaction of the TCR/CD3 complex with the antigen.

The T cell activation results in an increase of intracellular calcium. The association of other ligands presenting cells with antigen determinants surface of T cells involves an increase in the concentration of intracellular calcium and acts synergistically with the CD3 mediated events in the increasing activating T cell. One of these determinants, CD2, is considered to play a role both in cell to cell adhesion that in the activation of T cells. On the other hand CD4 and CD8, when bound to the antigen presenting cells, can produce an increase of intracellular calcium but not of T cell activation, as revealed by the production of interleukin-2 (IL-2) or from induction of cell proliferation. And interestingly, if the interaction with the antigen leads to the association of CD4 and CD8 with CD3, then the binding determinants on antigen-presenting cells induces T cell activation. Another surface molecule, CD54 (decay-accelerating factor DAF), does not increase the intracellular calcium per se, but the cross-linking of these molecules can induce T cell proliferation. Furthermore, the cross-linking of CD54 and CD3 results in an increase in calcium concentration induced by CD3 as well as the proliferation of T cells. Together with T cell activation, the activation of B cells is a necessary component of a proper immune function. Germinal centers in the follicular dendritic cells are probably the most important antigene presenting cells for B cells. They carry a large amount of antigen in the immune complexes containing complement. The antigen-antibody complexes are connected to follicular dendritic cells via complement and Fc receptors. This complex of macromolecules is incorporated in the ISCOMs (immunostimulating complexes), corpuscles linked to the membrane coated with immune complexes, which are released into the intercellular space, where the B cells are joined. The i Interaction of ISCOMs bounded antigen with the B cell is incremented because the proteins of the surface of B cells interact with both the antigenic determinants and the complement factors. This cross-linking of surface receptors of B cells leads to activation of the B cell. The involvement of complement factors can lead to the formation of terminal complement complex, which apparently did not cause any damage. The terminal complement complexes can lead to a release of inflammation mediators and mild edema. This intratonsillar edema facilitates the dispersion of ISCOMs and increases the chance of contact with B cells and their activation. B cells are further activated by helper T cells of tonsil via cell to cell contact and then the antigen presented to B-cells is further processed by them and thus presented to T cells in the context of class II molecules of human leukocyte antigen (HLA).

Together with the cell to cell interactions the activation of immune system is mediated by cytokines. At least 19 different cytokines are found in the tonsils of patients with infectious mononucleosis, or recurrent tonsillitis [6]. Cytokines are easily found in all areas of surface epithelium of the germinal center. The IL-2 is well known for its ability to increase the lymphocyte activation. The follicular dendritic cells induce the production of IL-6 and the clonal proliferation of T cells. Cytokines are also involved in the regulation of the production of IL-1, in the change of immunoglobulins in all IgG subclasses, in the production of IgA and induction of the Bcl-2 gene, which prevents the apoptosis of B immune activated lymphocytes.

The formation of an appropriate immune response, therefore, depends on a myriad of complex interactions between cryptic epithelial cells, macrophages, interdigitating cells, follicular dendritic cells, T cells, B cells and cytokines. The successful interactions lead to the production of activated B cells, which enter the bloodstream and at the same time are associated with the glandular tissue and the lamina propria of the epithelium of the upper respiratory tract [7] or differ locally in producing immunoglobulins cells. The IgA is the main immunoglobulin produced in the mucosa-associated lymphoid tissue (MALT) and in the areas of the upper respiratory tract is favored the production of IgA 1. In tonsils and adenoids, as in the rest of the MALT, are prevalent the IgG immunocytes and IgA-producing cells are around the 30% -35%. The IgA is a dimer, whose molecules are linked by a chain J [7].

In tonsils, adenoids unlike, dimeric IgA do not increase the range of secretory passage through the epithelium. While both IgA and IgG antibodies in the secretions pass directly through a link with pharyngeal epithelial cells. This is incremented by inflammation.

The infection leads to chronic and recurrent tonsillar hyperplasia and /or nodularity. Morphologic features include expansion of lymphoid follicles and prominent germinal centers formation, with intact mantle zone and mixture of cell types including B lymphocytes and T lymphocytes as well as histiocytes and plasma cells. Polymorphonuclear can be found within the epithelium and as aggregates within the crypts along with bacteria. Furthermore, multinucleated giant cells may occur during viral related infections.

Chronic inflammation initially involves an increase of reticular epithelialium. Later, however, the crypts become coated by squamous epithelium, devoid of M cells, which facilitate the entry of the antigen [8]. This can lead to a reduction in the amount of processed antigen for presentation to T cells. In addition, patients with tonsillar focal infection have a minor amount of tonsil follicular dendritic cells in the lymphoepithelial symbiosis. Since multiple interactions are necessary for proper T-cell response, the reduced antigen presentation may result in the suppression of the immune response. It has been shown that the suboptimal T cell signaling involves a partial activation and that partially activated T cells can produce cell surface receptors for cytokines but cannot proliferate. Such partial activation may currently lead to tolerance, inhibition of responsiveness and defective production of IL-2.

Bernstein & al. [9] have shown the decreased production of IL-2 in 34 patients who underwent adenoidectomy or adenotonsillectomy. In these patients, it was found that T cells of adenoids weakly support the production of B cells of the major isotopes of immunoglobulins. This was attributed to the reduction of the production of IL-2, in response to stimulation of both mitogens and specific antigens, by means of lymphocytes of adenoid and tonsil, in comparison with peripheral blood lymphocytes. Interestingly this reduction in the production of IL-2 was observed in the context of a very spontaneous lymphoproliferative activity. The authors suggested that the continuous bottom stimulation of tonsillar and adenoidal lymphocytes could lead to an increase in non-stimulated proliferative activity and a decrease of the response to specific antigenic challenges.

Even Koch and Brodsky [10] examined lymphocyte activation in patients with chronic tonsillitis. Noticed a decreased of proliferative response to stimulation by H. influenzae type B and S. pyogenes in the pathological tonsils than normal. In addition, after stimulation, the death rate of tonsillar lymphocytes was accelerated. Their observation suggests that the lymphocytes of pathologic tonsils become refractory or tolerant to immune activation by certain pathogens associated with chronic tonsillitis. This result was further supported and extended by other Authors who have examined the response of the tonsillar and peripheral blood lymphocytes to mitogen and antigenic stimulation. They found that, while the basal mitogenic activity was high, the response to stimulation in these two lymphocyte populations was weakened. This reduction in response was attributed to the continuous release of immunosuppressive factors, and the resumption of the proliferative response after tonsillectomy.

So in certain situations hyperplastic tonsils can be seen as immunocompromised organs that may reduce the total efficacy of the local immune system. Patients with recurrent tonsillitis are also deficient in B cells, perhaps for a decrease of IL-2 above mentioned or other additional changes in the profiles of the lymphokines produced by antigen-presenting cells and T cell subsets. Such changes may lead to a reduced retention of B-cell clones memory and a reduced production of secretory IgA.

This was evidenced by the reduced generation of B cells expressing the J chain in children with recurrent tonsillitis. Another important cell in the immune response is the neutrophil, which engulfs and destroys opsonized microorganisms. Chronic infections are acting negatively on neutrophil chemotactic function. The neutrophil function was studied in 17 patients between the ages of 4 and 11 years with chronic tonsillitis and adenoid hypertrophy. In such patients, chemotaxis was significantly lower compared to controls. The evaluation repeated 10 days after surgery showed no significant differences between the two groups, but the increase in the chemotactic response of neutrophil function after surgery was significant compared to preoperative values [11].

The chronic effect of adenotonsillectomy on immunoglobulins was studied at tonsil and peripheral blood. Several changes are induced by chronic, and some may be related to the presence of bacteria typically observed in adenotonsillar infections. As already stated, IgG and IgA are the primary antibodies produced in response to antigenic challenge, however is to be noted that the cells producing IgD are more prevalent in the MALT that in the gut associated lymphoid tissue [12]. This can achieve the stimulation of B-cell reserve, which express IgD, by H. influenzae and M. catarrhalis. These bacteria, which frequently colonize the upper aerodigestive tract, produce a binder IgD factor that has a cruciate connection with the IgD and with the molecules of class I human leukocyte antigen (HLA). This determines a polyclonal stimulation of the proliferation of B cells and results in an increased production of IgD and a preferential production of secretory IgA1 (SIgA1) above the production of IgA2.

The production of IgD and the preferential production of IgA1 have important implications for the local immune response. First, IgD cannot act as secretory immunoglobulin. So the cells directed to differentiate in the production of these immunoglobulins are actually being removed from the immune globuline-producer cellular pool. Secondly, the H. influenzae produces a protease that cleaves IgA1. Even St. pneumoniae and Neisseria meningitidis produce this protease. Thus these bacteria, which are often found in patients with chronic adenotonsillitis, have developed both a mechanism for guiding the antibody production to the IgA1 and a mechanism for cleaving this product with specific protease [13].

These modifications of immunoglobulin may be related to the common finding of immunoglobulin levels increased in the peripheral blood of patients with chronic tonsillitis. Significant elevations of IgG, IgA, IgM and IgE were found in patients with chronic tonsillitis. After tonsillectomy, these values return to normal [14]. This apparent paradox of increased immunoglobulin levels in patients with chronic infection can be explained by the studies discussed above on T and B cell. Given the constant stimulation of the immune system in patients with chronic adenotonsillitis, there is a bottom elevation of mitotic activity and antibody production. However, in response to stimulation by specific bacteria, the production above this baseline level is limited, as shown by the decrease of the activity of both mitogenic tonsillar lymphocytes and of those in the peripheral blood. Can also be a concomitant inability to increase the production of specific antibodies in response to specific infectious agents.

Kurono & al. [15] have illustrated the latter point by examining the levels of sIgA and the adherence of S. pyogenes cells in the nasal mucosa. Secretory IgA inhibit bacterial adherence to mucosal cells attaching to the surface and directly interfering with bacterial adherence to the epithelium of the antigenic component of the surface of the bacterium. In their study of 29 patients with chronic sinusitis the Authors showed high levels of sIgA compared to 25 controls. Nevertheless the bacterial adherence to the nasal mucosa was increased in patients with chronic sinusitis. It appears from these results that, in spite of the immune system can produce a great quantity of immunoglobulins, there may still be a decreased activity in response to specific antigens. A similar situation may exist in patients with chronic tonsillitis, but lack specific data.

The previous discussion emphasizes the multiple immune defects that may be present in patients with chronic tonsillitis. It may be noted that in these patients may present a cycle of infection which involves epithelial modifications responsible for decreased antigen presentation and immunity function which in turn lead to further infection. Other influences can further reduce the immune response. What factors are the causative agents and if are simple or associated factors has not been fully delineated.

3. Patients and methods

A total of 13 patients with psoriasis and recurrent tonsillitis subjected to tonsillectomy in the Department of ENT-Maxillofacial Surgery, San Giovanni Bosco Hospital, Turin, Italy, between March 2003 and August 2010 were enrolled in this study (Group 1). In addition, 9 patients with recurrent tonsillitis and without psoriasis subjected to tonsillectomy between June 2002 and September 2010 were enrolled in this study (Group 2). The diagnosis of psoriasis was confirmed by typical clinical findings and histopathological examination. The data were retrospectively reviewed to assess the epidemiological and clinical features.

Patients with psoriasis (Group 1) were further divided into two subgroups: patients without improvement of the psoriasis symptomatology (subgroup A, 4 patients) and patients with prolonged or temporary improvement of psoriasis symptomatology after tonsillectomy (subgroup B, 9 patients).

Eligibility requirements for both groups included a diagnosis of recurrent tonsillitis with none of the following other conditions: clinical history of allergy (alimentary, cutaneous or respiratory tract allergies), chronic respiratory pathologies (nasal septum deviation, hypertrophic rhinopathy, asthma, chronic sinusitis), surgical or clinical rhinopharyngeal and oral treatments (adenoidectomy, nasal polyps surgery, periodontal or peritonsillar abscesses drainage, dental or periodontal surgery).

Eligibility requirements for psoriasis group included a diagnosis of psoriasis made by a dermatologist, their disease course was followed for at least 2 years and their disease severity assessed by the Psoriasis Area and Severity Index (PASI). PASI is the standard method for evaluating changes in the extent and activity of this disease [16]. Improvement was evaluated according to at least 50% PASI score reduction. A PASI score reduction of at least 50% (PASI 50) is considered as clinically meaningful improvement [17].

The participants were evaluated clinically at study entry and after every 6 months.

The diagnosis of recurrent tonsillitis and eligibility for tonsillectomy was made according with the Italian Guidelines on the clinical and organisational appropriateness of tonsillectomy and adenoidectomy [18,19].

National guidelines issued in 2003 restricted the surgical option mainly to: children with significant obstructive apnea (adenotonsillectomy), children with recurrent otitis media and ventilation-tube placement or with chronic/recurrent sinusitis and failure of appropriate antibiotic therapy (adenoidectomy), children and adults with severe acute recurrent tonsillitis (tonsillectomy).

In those Guidelines it is suggested that tonsillectomy be limited to children and adults with recurrent acute bacterial tonsillitis of proven severity, meeting the following criteria:

–Five episodes of tonsillitis per year;

–Episodes that are disabling and prevent normal functioning; and

–Symptoms lasting at least 12 months.

The patients were all examined for tonsillar remnants at the end of the study and no tonsillar remnants could be detected in any patient of the study after the surgical intervention.

There were not alcohol drinkers. Each case was characterized by age, presenting signs and symptoms, and mean duration of clinical symptoms antedating clinical diagnosis and tonsillectomy. The patients had a full physical examination, complete blood counts and clinical laboratory tests including leucocyte count.

The number and duration of recurrent tonsillitis episodes as well as response to antibiotic treatment and history of medical conditions were recorded. Such clinical informations gathered on each patient were further outlined by considering available medical records, parents report and, when possible, by contacting each respective attending physician.

After a period of clinical examination and data recording, patients underwent tonsillectomy. Tonsils were removed by dissection and haemostasis was controlled with suction cautery, pressure and/or suture ligature. Patients follow-up revealed no post-operative complications.

Tonsils from both psoriatic and non psoriatic groups were collected, washed in buffered saline, measured along the three dimensions and immediately processed by conventional methods within half an hour after surgery.

In particular, perpendicular sections to the long axis of each tonsil were fixed in 10% neutral-buffered formalin, routinely processed for histology and stained with haematoxylin and eosin, periodic acid-Schiff (PAS) and Weigert van Gieson. The following parameters were recorded for the entire tonsillar area: surface and cryptic epithelial changes, follicles, subepithelial and interfollicular compartments.

On the contrary, small fragments (5-mm-thick) immediately collected after removal from the surface of each tonsil were fixed in 2% phosphate-buffered glutaraldehyde, post-fixed in osmium tetroxide, dehydrated with increasing concentrations of ethanol, dried in a critical-point apparatus under CO_2, and examined in a Hitachi emission field scanning electron microscope (SEM) (Hitachi Ltd., Tokyo, Japan) at 25 kV. The morphology of surface and cryptic epithelium, and specialized surface cells was analysed.

Light and SEM examinations were blinded performed without knowledge of the clinical history and patient's condition.

4. Results

The 13 patients with psoriasis - 6 males and 7 females - aged 9 to 46 years were followed up 2 to 5 years after tonsillectomy. The subgroup A consisted of 1 male and 3 female patients suffering of guttate (2 patients) and chronic plaque psoriasis (2 patients). The subgroup B consisted of 5 males and 4 females suffering of guttate (6 patients) and chronic plaque psoriasis (3 patients). Duration of psoriasis varied from 5 to 24 years in subgroup A and from 4 to 13 years in subgroup B. Improvement duration in the subgroup B varied from 6 months to 5 years. The 9 patients without psoriasis - 1 male and 5 females - aged 9 to 35 years.

Clinical data regarding patients with psoriasis and recurrent tonsillitis (Group 1), subgroups A and B are reported in Table 1 and Table 2 respectively, whereas table 3 shows clinical data of the patients with recurrent tonsillitis and without psoriasis (Group 2).

Patients with psoriasis and recurrent tonsillitis Group1, Subgroup A (No improvement after tonsillectomy) Improvement: absent or < 50% improvement of PASI score							
Patients	**Sex**	**Age**	**Number of annual tonsillitis**	**Duration of psoriasis**	**Follow-up**	**Type of psoriasis**	**Improvement duration / PASI score improvement**
1	F	46	8	24 years	4 years	Guttate psoriasis	18 months 30%
2	F	31	5	22 years	5 years	Chronic plaque psoriasis	No improvement
3	F	9	5	5 years	2 year	Chronic plaque psoriasis	No improvement
4	M	11	6	7 years	5 years	Guttate psoriasis	No improvement

Table 1. Clinical data of the patients with psoriasis and recurrent tonsillitis with no improvement after tonsillectomy: Subgroup A of Group 1.

Patients with psoriasis and recurrent tonsillitis Group 1, Subgroup B (Improvement after tonsillectomy) Improvement: = or "/> 50% improvement of PASI score							
Patients	**Sex**	**Age**	**Number of annual tonsillitis**	**Duration of psoriasis**	**Follow-up**	**Type of psoriasis**	**Improvement duration / PASI score improvement**
1	F	35	5	7 years	4 years	Guttate psoriasis	4 years/ 50%
2	M	12	6	8 years	3 years	Chronic plaque psoriasis	6 months 90%
3	M	22	7	7 years	2 Years	Chronic plaque psoriasis	12 months 50%
4	M	10	6	6 years	2 years	Guttate psoriasis	6 months 75%
5	M	12	7	5 years	3 years	Guttate psoriasis	12 months 75%
6	M	9	5	5 years	5 years	Guttate psoriasis	3 years 90%
7	F	11	7	5 years	5 years	Guttate psoriasis	18 months 75%
8	F	10	5	4 years	3 years	Chronic plaque psoriasis	6 months 100%
9	F	18	5	13 years	5 years	Guttate psoriasis	5 years 50%

Table 2. Clinical data of the patients with psoriasis and recurrent tonsillitis with improvement after tonsillectomy: Subgroup B of Group 1.

Patients with recurrent tonsillitis and without psoriasis			
Patients	**Sex**	**Number of annual tonsillitis**	**Age**
1	M	7	13
2	F	6	12
3	F	6	18
4	M	6	29
5	M	5	11
6	F	5	10
7	F	7	9
8	F	5	35
9	M	5	18

Table 3. Clinical data of the patients with recurrent tonsillitis and without psoriasis: Group 2.

Clinical findings demonstrated clear differences between psoriatic and non-psoriatic group, the former showing further differences between subgroup with long-term or short-term improvement of psoriasis symptoms (subgroup B) and subgroup with no-improvement after tonsillectomy (subgroup A).

Psoriasis had long term improvement (PASI = OR < 50%) after tonsillectomy in two out of the eight patients (25%) with guttate psoriasis and had a short-time improvement in four patient (50%). Three out of five patients with chronic plaque psoriasis (60%) had a short-time improvement, two (40%) were unchanged.

On the other hand, light microscopy and SEM findings showed minimal differences between the control and both psoriatic subgroup A and B.

Histology of tonsils revealed well-known morphological features of reactive and hyper-plastic pattern in both psoriatic and non-psoriatic groups. Secondary follicles with well-defined germinal centres and mantle zones, irregular and enlarged follicles and florid follicular hyperplasia were usually observed. Clear follicular expansion and irregularity as well as evident infiltration of lymphoid cells in the tonsillar crypt epithelium, along with irregularity of the epithelial wavy basal membrane and epithelial basal profile were noted in two cases from psoriatic subgroup B: case 6 and case 9.

Interstitial fibrosis along with a dense collagen matrix seemed more evident in both A and B psoriatic subgroups compared to non-psoriatic patients and were sometimes associated with a variable degree of stromal oedema and haemorrhages. A fine small blood vessels network was clearly observed in both groups beneath the epithelial surface and in association with the reticulated epithelium as finger-like projections surrounded by connective tissue, with hyperaemia and extravasated red blood cells. Blood vessels thickening or microscopic features of vasculitis were not observed in either groups.

Tonsillar crypt epithelium showed cellular degeneration, variable degree of thickness and intercellular spongiosis or micro-vescicular formation, with no histological distinctive pattern or significant quantitative differences between psoriatic and non-psoriatic patients. Both groups showed some dilated and pseudocystic crypts lined by squamous epithelium and filled with squamous debris along with a mixture of lymphocytes, neutrophils and desquamated epithelial cells. Bacterial aggregates were sometimes observed near or within the crypt lumen in both groups.

Scanning electron microscopy correlated with histology and revealed the surface epithelium consisting of squamous and sometimes keratinized cells in an irregular pattern of microridges and sometimes rod-like elements, referring to bacteria, adhering to the epithelium, in both psoriatic and non-psoriatic patients (Fig.1). A fine meshed and sometimes cerebroid-like net of the epithelial surface was observed. Specialized surface cells with short microvilli were noted close to lymphocytes or macrophages. Lymphoid cells were frequently observed near the crypt lumen along with surface cellular debris, detached epithelial cells and scattered bacteria (Fig. 2).

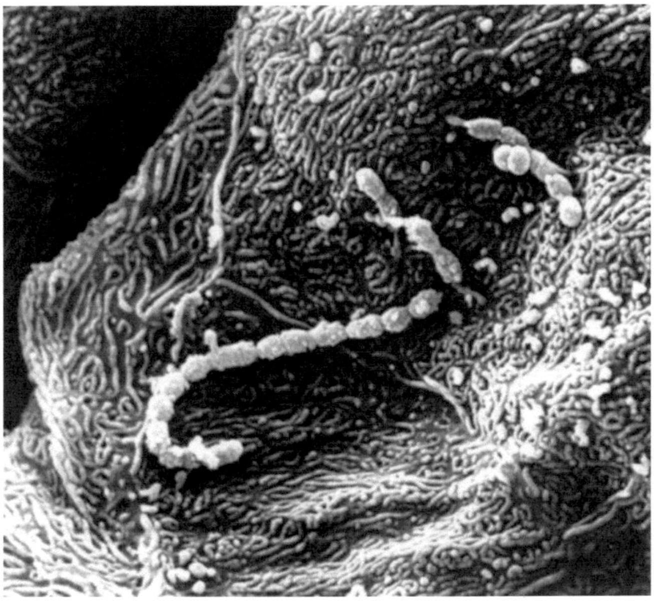

Figure 1. Particular of the surface tonsillar epithelium(patient 4 of Group 1, Subgroup A): rod-like elements, referring to bacteria, adhering to the epithelium, in a more or less intact area (scanning electron micrograph, x1000).

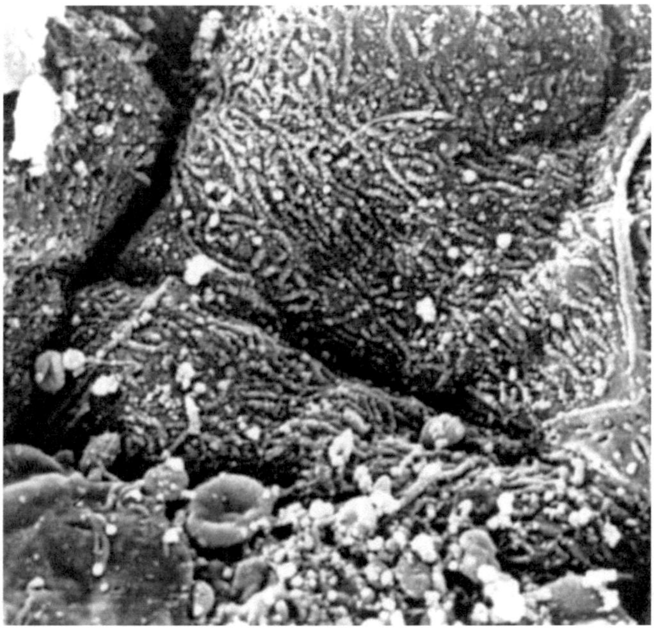

Figure 2. Particular of the surface tonsillar epithelium (patient 6 of Group 1, Subgroup B): accentuated reticulation of epithelial elements; crypts are hard to find, often masked by debris, mucus and epithelial desquamation (scanning electron micrograph, x1000)

http://dx.doi.org/10.5772/55978

5. Discussion

Recently was postulated that psoriasis is a genetic based chronic cutaneous inflammatory disorder, involving several genes encoding proteins involved in epidermal differentiation and immune, inflammatory and pathogenic responses, in combination with microbial environmental factors. The importance of the microbial environment is fundamental to demonstrate the correlation between genetic ground and clinical manifestation, because these agents may function as triggers for immunological dysregulated responses, especially in a particular context in which there is an impaired capacity of barrier organs to regulate microbial flora and prevent entrance of bacteria, viruses and fungi [20].

The association between streptococcal infections and guttate psoriasis or plaque psoriasis and has been known for a long time and is well-documented.

The mechanisms, however, are still a matter of investigation and several findings indicate a possible role for various bacterial proteins and/or toxins serving as superantigens.

Psoriasis exacerbation has been linked with skin and/or gut colonization by Staphylococcus aureus, Malassezia, and Candida albicans. The role, if any, of viruses (papillomaviruses, HIV, and endogenous retroviruses) present in lesional skin is at present unknown. The use of various drugs, such as lithium, β-blockers, antimalarial agents, nonsteroidal anti-inflammatory drugs, and angiotensin-converting enzyme inhibitors, has also been associated with induction or worsening of disease in psoriatic patients [21].

The triggering of guttate psoriasis was initially associated with Lancefield group A streptococci (S pyogenes), but streptococci of groups C and G have also been isolated from the tonsils of patients with guttate psoriasis. Group A (C and G) streptococci express one of several antigenically distinct M proteins on their surface; however, no association has yet been found between particular M serotypes and the triggering of guttate psorisis by group A streptococci [22,23].

Honig [24] found an association between perianal streptococcal dermatitis and guttate psoriasis, while Rasi & al. [25] found the association between perianal streptococcal dermatitis and plaque-type psoriasis.

Based on epidemiological data McFadden & al. [26] postuled the natural selection of psoriasis, whose immunological pathways may confer protection against mortality during epidemics of invasive streptococcal infections, heightened efficiency in internalizing and allowing carriage of streptococci as well as predisposition to the development of psoriasis.

The first report that the onset of guttate psoriasis is often preceded by throat infections with b-haemolytic is due to Winfield in 1916 [27]. The link between psoriasis and streptococcal infection is probably explained by the 'superantigen theory'. The streptococcus carries a protein called the M-protein which allows it to act as a superantigen. Superantigens are bacterial or viral products that can bypass normal immunological pathways and cause powerful stimulation of the immune system. This results in the production of T-lymphocytes (white blood cells) which have been shown to be central to the development of psoriasis.

Streptococcal throat infections are related to the incidence of psoriasis onset is also highest between the ages of 11 and 20 years.

In children, the first manifestation of psoriasis is commonly drop- like with sudden onset after an infection of the upper airways. The guttate psoriasis is localized predominantly in the exposed parts of the body, such as the face and limbs. The lesion has a diameter of about 1-3 cm, in color from pink to red, with the scales overlying gray or silver. The frequency of this clinical variety, characterized by acute onset and guttate lesions, decreases with increasing age, so as to become rare in the adult, when the predominant form is plaque psoriasis.

The plaque psoriasis, as opposed to the drop-like form, prefers the surfaces of the skin at bony eminences, such as the knuckles, elbows and knees. Approximately 30-50% of children with psoriasis has a family history of the disease. The psoriasis is in fact more often associated with antigen CW6 of class I HLA. The principal gene of susceptibility to psoriasis appears to resides on chromosome 6, which is just the home of the HLA complex HLA I and II. But probably many other genes are involved, as there are also external environmental influences, which recently were shown to be very important.

Streptococcal throat infections are most common around puberty and the incidence of psoriasis onset. Psoriasis is not uncommon in pediatric age group, becouse 27% of cases manifest before the age of 16 years; moreover, psoriasis represents 4.1% of all dermatoses seen in children under the age of 16 years [28].

Literature data on juvenile psoriasis are shown in table 4.

Author	N° of patients	Male:female ratio	Peak age of onset (years)	Infection precipitating factor	Plaque type incidence
Morris 2001 [29]	1262	1:1.14	8	-	34%
Kumar 2004 [30]	419	1.09:1	6-14	6.6%	60.6%
Kim 2010 [31]	30	1:2.33	8-11	43.4%	63%
Seyhan 2006 [32]	61	1:1.65	6-11	14.8%	54.1%
Dhar 2011 [33]	419	1.25:1	6-10	28.5%	60.6%
Kwon 2012 [34]	358	1.06:1	10-11	-	67%

Table 4. Literature data on juvenile psoriasis

In a previous retrospective study, about 30% of patients with chronic psoriasis reported that they had noted worsening of their disease in association with sore throat [35]. The same Author successively observed a significant exacerbation of chronic plaque psoriasis only if streptococci were isolated and the patients were assessed 4 days or later after the onset of sore throat. No difference was observed between groups A, C or G streptococci in this respect.

Consecutively psoriasis patients should be encouraged to report sore throat to their physician and that early treatment of streptococcal throat infections might be beneficial in psoriasis[36].

According to Camisa [37]: "In general new onset guttate psoriasis related to streptococcal infection involutes rapidly within a four week period with antibiotic treatment. In patients

http://dx.doi.org/10.5772/55978

with chronic psoriasis who develop a guttate exacerbation, empiric treatment with antibiotics is indicated".

Furthermore Farber [38] stated: "prevention and early treatment with appropriate antibiotics administered at the onset of upper respiratory infections in children with psoriasis may be able to block the appearance of acute guttate psoriasis".

A study confirms the strong association between prior infection with Streptococcus pyogenes and guttate psoriasis but suggests that the ability to trigger guttate psoriasis is not serotype specific [23].

The usefulness of early treatment of streptococcal infections for childhood psoriasis was demonstrated with a study about relationship between anti-streptolysin O (ASO) titers and the clinical features of psoriasis

The Authors also stated that the childhood psoriasis patients with high ASO titers had guttate psoriasis more frequently than patients with normal ASO titers. In children with plaque-type psoriasis, psoriasis area and severity index score was increased in the high ASO titer group than normal ASO titer group [31].

In literature was also stated the efficacy of tonsillectomy in the treatment of psoriasis [39-42].

Literature data on the employment of tonsillectomy for psoriasis improvement are shown in table 5. Unfortunately for some work has not been possible to find the full bibliographic data.

Wilson et al. (2003) [55] evaluated 27 retrospective and 28 prospective uncontrolled studies on effect of tonsillectomy on psoriasis and founded 32% and 53% cleared percentages respectively.

Relapse of the psoriasis often occurs within 2 years of tonsil removal, probably due to colonization by streptococci of other lymphoid tissues in the upper respiratory tract.

Hone & al. in 1996 [40] investigated 13 patients with either recurrent guttate psoriasis or chronic plaque psoriasis exacerbated by tonsillitis. In this group, psoriasis cleared completely after tonsillectomy in five of six patients with guttate psoriasis and two of seven with chronic plaque psoriasis.

Rosenberg & al. [50] reported clearing of psoriasis in nine of 14 patients (all of whom had evidence of streptococcal colonisation) following tonsillectomy.

McMillin & al. [41] found that two children with recurrent streptococcal pharyngitis or tonsillitis complicated by recurrent guttate psoriasis were completely free of psoriasis 16 months after adenotonsillectomy.

Despite those assertions, a recent Cochrane review [56] concluded: "although it is well known that guttate psoriasis may be precipitated by streptococcal infection, there is no firm evidence to support the use of antibiotics either in the management of established guttate psoriasis or in preventing the development of guttate psoriasis following streptococcal sore throat. Although both antibiotics and tonsillectomy have frequently been advocated for patients with

Author	N° of patients	Age	Type of psoriasis	Cleared or improved rate	Follow-up
Kogon 1960 [43]	-	-	-	-	-
Whyte 1964 [44]	3	15-23	Guttate	~100% cleared	1 year
Cepicka 1967 [45]	92	-	-	61% cleared	2-5 years
Stukalenko 1967 [46]	3	-	-	-	-
Lukovskii 1970 [47]	57	-	-	89% improved	-
Nyfors 1976 [39]	74	4-33	Vulgaris	32% cleared	7-204 months
Saita 1979 [48]	2	7-11	Guttate	~100% cleared	-
Hone 1996 [40]	13	6-28	6 Guttate 7 Chronic Plaque	83% Guttate cleared 28% Chronic plaque cleared	6-52 months
Kataura 1996 [49]	35	-	Vulgaris	49% cleared	3 months
Rosenberg 1998 [50]	14	-	-	64% cleared	-
McMillin 1999 [41]	2	5-11	1 Guttate 1 Severe	~100% cleared	16 months
Ozawa 1999 [42]	385	-	Generalized pustular	16% cleared	-
Takahara 2001 [51]	7	9-46	-	42% cleared	2-9 years
Prasad 2005 [52]	13	5-36	-	75% improvement SAPASI score	-
Diluvio 2006 [53]	3	21-33	Ch. Plaque	~100% cleared	3 years
Thorleifsdottir 2012 [54]	29	19-54	-	86% cleared (30-90%)	2 years

Table 5. Literature data on tonsillectomy for psoriasis treatment.

recurrent guttate psoriasis or chronic plaque psoriasis, there is to date no good evidence that either intervention is beneficial".

Thorleifsdottir & al. [57] suggested that psoriatic patients after tonsillectomy has at least a temporary beneficial effect on chronic psoriasis, and is associated with a striking reduction in the frequency of circulating skin-homing CD8+ T cells that are specific for peptides with amino acid sequences that are present in both streptococcal M-proteins and human keratins. These amino acid sequences might therefore represent antigen determinants that are relevant in psoriasis. In a successive study the same Author [54] stated that there is a close correlation between the degree of clinical improvement in individual patients and reduction in the frequency of peptide-reactive skin-homing T cells in their circulation and therefore tonsillectomy may have a beneficial effect on chronic psoriasis because the palatine tonsils generate effector T cells that recognize keratin determinants in the skin. According to this Author: "identification of circulating T cells that respond to homologous M protein and keratin determinants in patients with treatment-induced remission may help to identify primary autoepitopes that might be targeted for highly specific immunotherapy for psoriasis".

A recent European expert group consensus [58] stated that: "in cases where there is a positive streptococcal swab and more than three recurrent infections, tonsillectomies are indicated for patients with plaque or guttate psoriasis".

Perhaps, according to Sigurdardottir [59]: "Some patients with recalcitrant guttate or chronic plaque psoriasis, particularly those with early-onset psoriasis that is exacerbated by streptococcal tonsillitis appear to have long-term remissions following tonsillectomy".

Some authors have highlighted the differences from the histological point of view between the tonsils of patients who achieved an improvement of psoriasis after tonsillectomy, compared to the tonsils of patients who did not obtain this improvement [51]. The above mentioned differences are related to the expansion of the T cell-nodules area and the increasing of the number of apoptotic cells in tonsil from patients with psoriasis compared to those with recurrent tonsillitis. The Authors suggested that histological evaluation may be helpful in estimating the effectiveness of tonsillectomy.

6. Conclusion

Association between psoriasis and streptococcal pharyngitis has been recognized for many years. To explain the possible association between drop elements of the psoriasis and infections of the pharynx by Streptococcus is necessary to focuses on immunology of the skin.

In the skin there are 3 types of antigen-presenting cells:

a. the Langerhans cells

b. the dermal dendrocytes

c. the tissue macrophages

Their function is to attack the proteins, to insert their fragments (epitopes) in complex MHC I and II, which are present on the cell surface and to present these antigens to T-cell receptors.An activation signal occurs when the B7 on the surface of antigen presenting cells binds to the CD28 receptor of T cell The thus activated T cell begins to produce cytokines. In psoriasis T cells of the skin are primarily CD8 + cells in the epidermis and CD4 + in the dermis. Cytokines are represented by interleukin 2 (IL-2) that activate other T cells and the gamma interferon, which enhances the expression of cell surface antigens of the MHC [60].

Superantigens are presented by antigen presenting cells without the need of a preparation and presentation in the MHC complex. The superantigens strep attach directly to the V region of the beta-2 CD4 + T cells, which preferably harbored in the skin. The stimulation of the superantigen activates more than 10% of all lymphocytes exposed, while the conventional antigens, expressed on the T cell receptors, stimulates only about 1 in 10,000 T cells.

These activated T cells, mainly CD4 +, they release a large number of cytokines, including IL-2, interferon gamma and growth factors, which attract T cells and CD8 + T cells of the epidermis. The stimulation of the population of suprabasal keratinocytes, by the cells transiently multiplying, determines an hyperproliferation, increases the resistance to apoptosis and increases the expression of keratin, including the keratin 14 of the skin. Recent information suggests that there is a strong homology between the keratin 14 of the skin and M-6 of Streptococcus.

So there can be a large population of T cells (V beta-2, CLA +), that lodge in the skin, which are activated by the superantigen Streptococcus; between these some T cells responding to the antigen M-6 of the Streptococcus, that cross-reacts with cutaneous keratinocytes 14. This cascade of events may be the cause of the injury thickened and red, that dermatologists and pediatricians recognize as guttate psoriasis.

In short, the processes that lead to the appearance of guttate psoriasis in susceptible individuals after Streptococcus infection can be done in two stages.

The streptococcal superantigen in genetically susceptible individuals actives most of the CD4 + T cells that lodge in the skin, as the target organ. These activated T cells, that lodge in the dermis and epidermis, they release IL-2, gamma-interferon and other cytokines, which attract lymphocytes CD8 +, which induce cell transient amplification. The resulting explosion of hyperproliferative activity is the basis of guttate lesions. The epidermis hyperproliferative activity also increases the expression of keratins, such as keratin 14. The cycle can be perpetuated and exacerbated by T cells, that are specifically sensitized to the M protein of Streptococcus that shows a strong homology with the keratin 14 of the skin.

There is other evidence of the immunological basis of psoriasis:

a. bone marrow transplants in patients with psoriasis cause psoriasis spent recipients, while bone marrow from normal individuals may induce a remission of the disease;

b. similar results were obtained experimentally in mice with severe combined immunodeficiency;

c. all substances effective in the treatment of psoriasis, act on T cells (cyclosporine, rapamycin, corticosteroids, retinoids, vitamin D and analogues, methotrexate).

Treatment outcomes of tonsillectomy were studied in 13 italian patients with psoriasis- 6 males and 5 females aged 9 to 46 years - followed up 2 to 5 years after tonsillectomy. There were 8 cases of guttate psoriasis and 5 cases of chronic plaque psoriasis. The PASI score improved for at least 50% for the entire follow-up period in two patients and in a short period (not inferior to 6 months) in 7 patients. A little improvement of PASI score (30%) was observed for 18 months in 1 patient. No change was found in the remaining 3 during follow-up period. Out of 9, whose skin lesions have improved, 4 were females and had a history of tonsillitis making skin lesions worse.

Light microscopy and SEM findings showed minimal differences between the control and both psoriatic subgroup A and B. At light microscopy examination, clear follicular expansion and irregularity as well as evident infiltration of lymphoid cells in the tonsillar crypt epithelium, along with irregularity of the epithelial wavy basal membrane and epithelial basal profile were noted in two cases from psoriatic subgroup B.

http://dx.doi.org/10.5772/55978

This preliminary report needs further investigation on a more large casuistry for conclusions validation. The paper is not intended to promote the tonsillectomy for the treatment of psoriasis, but try to contribute to the now confirmed conviction of the international literature on the relationship between psoriasis and streptococcal infection.

However, despite Cochrane review[56] conclusions, numerous reports indicate the improving role of tonsillectomy in some cases of psoriasis. The challenge of future research is the understanding of what kind of patients are susceptible to this improvement, in order to customize the use of the surgical treatment of tonsillectomy for patients with psoriasis and to better define the relationship between this disease and streptococcal infection.

Author details

Sebastiano Bucolo[1], Valerio Torre[2], Giuseppe Romano[3], Carmelo Quattrocchi[4], Filippo Farri[5], Maura Filidoro[6] and Claudio Caldarelli[1]

1 ENT–Maxillofacial Surgery Department, San Giovanni Bosco Hospital, Turin, Italy

2 Department of Pathology, San Donato Hospital, Arezzo, Italy

3 ENT Depepartment, Hospital of Milazzo, Milazzo, Italy

4 ENT Depepartment, University of Messina, Messina, Italy

5 ENT Depepartment, University of Novara, Novara, Italy

6 ENT Depepartment, University of Genova, Genova, Italy

References

[1] Surján L Jr. Immunohistochemical markers of tonsillar crypt epithelium. Acta Otolaryngol Suppl 1988;454:60-63.

[2] Jego G, Pascual V, Palucka AK, Banchereau J. Dendritic Cells Control B Cell Growth and Differentiation. In B Cell Trophic Factors and B Cell Antagonism in Autoimmune Disease. Curr Dir Autoimmun, Stohl W (ed), Basel, Karger 2005;vol 8, pp 124-139. doi: 10.1159/000082101.

[3] Kasenõnm P, Mesila I, Piirsoo A, Kull M, Mikelsaar M, Mikelsaar RH. Macroscopic oropharyngeal signs indicating impaired defensive function of palatine tonsils in adults suffering from recurrent tonsillitis. APMIS 2004;112: 248–256. doi: 10.1111/j.1600-0463.2004.apm11204-0504.x.

[4] Skibinski G, Skibinska A, James K. Tonsil stromal cell lines expressing follicular dendritic cell-like properties--isolation, characterization and interaction with B lymphocytes. Biochem Soc Trans 1997;25:233S.

[5] Steiniger B, Trabandt M, Barth PJ. The follicular dendritic cell network in secondary follicles of human palatine tonsils and spleens. Histochemistry and Cell Biology 2011;135:327-336. doi : 10.1007/s00418-011-0799-x.

[6] Andersson J, Abrams J, Björk L, Funa K, Litton M, Agren K, Andersson U. Concomitant in vivo production of 19 different cytokines in human tonsils. Immunology 1994;83:16-24.

[7] Brandtzaeg P, Jahnsen FL, Farstad IN. Immune functions and immunopathology of the mucosa of the upper respiratory pathways.? 1996;116(2):149-159.

[8] Kraehenbuhl JP, Neutra MR. Epithelial M cells: differentiation and function. Annu Rev Cell Dev Biol 2000;16:301-32.

[9] Bernstein JM, Ballow M, Rich G. Detection of intracytoplasmic cytokines by flow cytometry in adenoids and peripheral blood lymphocytes of children. Ann Otol Rhinol Laryngol 2001;110:442-446.

[10] Koch RJ, Brodsky L. Qualitative and quantitative immunoglobulin production by specific bacteria in chronic tonsillar disease. Laryngoscope 1995;105:42-48.

[11] Sennaroglu L, Onerci M, Hascelik G. The effect of tonsillectomy and adenoidectomy on neutrophil chemotaxis. Laryngoscope 1993;103:1349-1351.

[12] Farstad IN, Halstensen TS, Kvale D, Fausa O, Brandtzaeg P. Topographic distribution of homing receptors on B and T cells in human gut-associated lymphoid tissue: relation of L-selectin and integrin alpha 4 beta 7 to naive and memory phenotypes. Am J Pathol 1997;150:187-199.

[13] Kilian M, Reinholdt J, Lomholt H, Poulsen K, Frandsen EV. Biological significance of IgA1 proteases in bacterial colonization and pathogenesis: critical evaluation of experimental evidence. APMIS 1996;104:321-338.

[14] Ikincioğullari A, Doğu F, Ikincioğullari A, Eğin Y, Babacan E. Is immune system influenced by adenotonsillectomy in children? Int J Pediatr Otorhinolaryngol 2002;66:251-257.

[15] Kurono Y, Fujiyoshi T, Mogi G. Secretory IgA and bacterial adherence to nasal mucosal cells. Ann Otol Rhinol Laryngol 1989;98:273-277.

[16] Fredriksson T, Pettersson U. Severe psoriasis – oral therapy with a new retinoid. Dermatologica 1978;157:238–244.

[17] Carlin CS, Feldman SR, Krueger JG, Menter A, Krueger GG. A 50% reduction in the Psoriasis Area and Severity Index (PASI 50) is a clinically significant endpoint in the assessment of psoriasis. J Am Acad Dermatol 2004;50: 859–866.

[18] PNLG (Programma Nazionale Linee Guida) Document n. 4 The Italian National Program for Clinical Practice Guidelines. Italian Ministry of Health, National Institue of Health, Agency of Public Health, Lazio Region, LINCO Project 2003. http://www.snlg-iss.it/PNLG/LG/007tonsille/tonsillectomy.pdf.

[19] Materia E, Baglio G, Bellussi L, Marchisio P, Perletti L, Pallestrini E, Calia V. The clinical and organisational appropriateness of tonsillectomy and adenoidectomy-an Italian perspective. Int J Pediatr Otorhinolaryngol 2005;69:497–500. doi: 10.1016/j.ijporl.2004.11.016.

[20] Mattozzi C, AG Richetta, Cantisani C, L Macaluso, Calvieri S. Psoriasis: New insight about pathogenesis, role of barrier organ integrity, NLR/CATERPILLER family genes and microbial flora. Dermatol 2012;39:752-60. doi: 10.1111/j.1346-8138.2012.01606.x. Epub 2012 Giu 14.

[21] Fry L, Baker BS. Triggering psoriasis: the role of infections and medications. Clinics in Dermatology 2007;25:606–615. doi:10.1016/j.clindermatol.2007.08.015.

[22] Belew PW, Wannamaker LW, Johnson D, Rosenberg EW. Beta haemolytic streptococcal types associated with psoriasis. In Recent advances in streptococci and streptococcal diseases. Kimura K, Kotami S, Shiokawa Y. Editors. UK: Readbooks Ltd 1985, p. 334.

[23] Telfer NR, Chalmers RJ, Whale K, Colman G. The role of streptococcal infection in the initiation of guttate psoriasis, Arch Dermatol,1992;128:39-42.

[24] Honig PJ. Guttate psoriasis associated with perianal streptococcal disease. J Pediatr 1998;113: 1037 – 1039.

[25] Rasi A, Pour-Heidari N. Association between Plaque-Type Psoriasis and Perianal Streptococcal Cellulitis and Review of the Literature. Arch Iran Med 2009;12:591–594.

[26] McFadden JP, Baker BS, Powles AV, Fry L. Psoriasis and streptococci: the natural selection of psoriasis revisited. Br J Dermatol 2009;160:929–937. Doi: 10.1111/j.1365-2133.2009.09102.x.

[27] Winfield JM. Psoriasis as a sequel to acute inflammations of the tonsils: a clinical note, J Cutan Dis,1916;34: 441–443.

[28] Trueb RM. Therapies for childhood psoriasis, Curr Probl Dermatol,2009;38:137-159. Epub 2009 Jul 28.

[29] Morris A, Rogers M, Fischer G, Williams K. Childhood psoriasis: a clinical review of 1262 cases. Pediatr Dermatol 2001;18:188–198

[30] Kumar B, Jain R, Sandhu K, Kaur I, Handa S. Epidemiology of childhood psoriasis: a study of 419 patients from northern India. Int J Dermatol 2004;43:654-658.

[31] Kim SK, Kang HY, Kim YC, Lee E-S. Clinical comparison of psoriasis in Korean adults and children: correlation with serum anti-streptolysin O titers. Arch Dermatol Res 2010;302:295–299. doi 10.1007/s00403-009-1025-8.

[32] Seyhan M, Coskun BK, Saglam H, Özcan H, Karincaoĝlu Y. Psoriasis in childhood and adolescence: evaluation of demographic and clinical features. Pediatrics International 2006;48:525-530.doi:10.1111/j.1442-200X.2006.02270.x.

[33] Dhar S, Banerjee R, Agrawal N, Chatterjee S, Malakar R. Psoriasis in children: an insight. Indian J Dermatol 2011;56: 262–265. doi: 10.4103/0019-5154.82477.

[34] Kwon HH, Na SJ, Jo SJ, Youn JI. Epidemiology and clinical features of pediatric psoriasis in tertiary referral psoriasis clinic. J Dermatol 2012;39:260-264. doi: 10.1111/j. 1346-8138.2011.01452.x. Epub 2011 Dec 29.

[35] Gudjonsson JE, Kárason A, Antonsdóttir AA, Rúnarsdóttir EH, Gulcher JR, Stefánsson K, Valdimarsson H. HLA-Cw6- positive and HLA-Cw6-negative patients with psoriasis vulgaris have distinct clinical features. J Invest Dermatol 2002;118:362–365.

[36] Gudjonsson JE, Thorarinsson AM, Sigurgeirsson B, Kristinsson KG, Valdimarsson H. Streptococcal throat infections and exacerbation of chronic plaque psoriasis: a prospective study. British Journal of Dermatology 2003;149: 530–534.

[37] Camisa C. Psoriasis. Cambridge, Mass. Blackwell Scientific Publications Inc.,1994.

[38] Farber EM, Nall L. Guttate psoriasis. Cutis 1993;51:157–164.

[39] Nyfors A, Rasmussen PA, Lemholt K, Eriksen B. Improvement of recalcitrant psoriasis vulgaris after tonsillectomy. J Laryngol Otol 1976;90:789-794.

[40] Hone SW, Donnelly MJ, Powell F, Blayney AW. Clearance of recalcitrant psoriasis after tonsillectomy. Clin Otolaryngol 1996;21:546-547.

[41] McMillin BD, Maddern BR,Graham WR. A role for tonsillectomy in the treatment of psoriasis? Ear Nose Throat J 1999;78:155-158.

[42] Ozawa A, Ohkido M, Haruki Y, Kobayashi H, Ohkawara A, Ohno Y, Inaba Y, Ogawa H. Treatments of generalized pustular psoriasis: a multicenter study in Japan. J Dermatol 1999;26: 141-149.

[43] Kogon GK, Protopopov NI, Zel'din GS, Titar GM. The efficacy of tonsillectomy in patients with chronic tonsillitis and psoriasis. Vestn Rentgenol Radiol 1960;34:52-55.

[44] Whyte HJ & Baughman RD. Acute Guttate Psoriasis and Streptococcal Infection, Arch Dermatol,1964;89:350-356.

[45] Cepicka W, Tielsch R. Focal infections and Psoriasis vulgaris. Dermatol Wochenschr 1967;153:193-199.

[46] Stukalenko AA. Recovery from psoriasis after tonsillectomy. Vestn Otorinolaringol 1967;29:101-102.

[47] Lukovskiĭ LA, Nesterenko GB, Tytar' GM, Bashmakov GV. Immediate and remote results of tonsillectomy in chronic tonsillitis and psoriasis. Vestn Otorinolaringol 1970;32:23-26.

[48] Saita B, Ishii Y, Ogata K, Kikuchi I, Inoue S, Naritomi K. Two sisters with guttate psoriasis responsive to tonsillectomy: case reports with HLA studies. J Dermatol 1979;6:185-189.

[49] Kataura A, Tsubota H. Clinical analyses of focus tonsil and related diseases in Japan. Acta Otolaryngol Suppl 1996;523:161-164.

[50] Rosenberg EW, Skinner RB, Noah PW. Anti-infectious therapy in psoriasis. In: Psoriasis (Roenigk HH, Maibach HI, eds), 3rd edn. New York: Marcel Dekker 1998;373-379.

[51] Takahara M, Bandoh N, Imada M, Hayashi T, Nonaka S, Harabuchi Y. Efficacy of tonsillectomy on psoriasis and tonsil histology. Nihon Jibiinkoka Gakkai Kaiho 2001;104:1065-1070.

[52] Prasad V, Mani N, Suraliraj A, Burova K, Hoare TJ. Tonsillectomy for psoriasis: does it help? In (2006) British Association of Otolaryngologists Head and Neck Surgeons Summer Meeting, 7–8 September 2005, Edinburgh, Scotland, UK: general abstracts. The Journal of Laryngology & Otology 2005;120,e26.doi:10.1017/S0022215106001186.

[53] Diluvio L, Vollmer S, Besgen P, Ellwart JW, Chimenti S, Prinz JC. Identical TCR beta-Chain Rearrangements in Streptococcal Angina and Skin Lesions of Patients with Psoriasis Vulgaris. J Immunol 2006; 176: 7104-7111.

[54] Thorleifsdottir RH, Sigurdardottir SL, Sigurgeirsson B, Olafsson JH, Sigurdsson MI, Petersen H, Arnadottir S, Gudjonsson JE, Johnston A, Valdimarsson H. Improvement of Psoriasis after Tonsillectomy Is Associated with a Decrease in the Frequency of Circulating T Cells That Recognize Streptococcal Determinants and Homologous Skin Determinants, J Immunol,2012;188:5160-5165.doi:10.4049/jimmunol.1102834. http://www.jimmunol.org/content/188/10/5160.

[55] Wilson JK, Al-Suwaidan SN, Krowchuk D, Feldman SR. Treatment of psoriasis in children: is there a role for antibiotic therapy and tonsillectomy? Pediatr Dermatol 2003;20:11-5.

[56] Owen CM, Chalmers R, O'Sullivan T, Griffiths CEM. Antistreptococcal interventions for guttate and chronic plaque psoriasis. Cochrane Database of Systematic Reviews 2000, Issue 2. Art. No.: CD001976. DOI: 10.1002/14651858.CD001976.

[57] Thorleifsdottir RH, Johnston A, Sigurdardottir SL, Olafsson JH, Sigurgeirsson B, Petersen H, Gudjonsson JE, Valdimarsson H. The impact of tonsillectomy on patients with chronic plaque psoriasis - A controlled study, Journal of Investigative Dermatology,2009;129,SUPPL1 (S20).

[58] Ståhle M, Atakan N, Boehncke WH, Chimenti S, Daudén E, Giannetti A, Hoeger P, Joly P, Katsambas A, Kragballe K, Lambert J, Ortonne J-P, Prinz J C, Puig L, Seyger

M, Strohal R, Van De Kerkhoff P, Sterry W. Juvenile psoriasis and its clinical management: a European expert group consensus. JDDG: Journal der Deutschen Dermatologischen Gesellschaft 2010;8:812–818.doi: 10.1111/j.1610-0387.2010.07507.x

[59] Sigurdardottir SL, Thorleifsdottir RH, Valdimarsson H, Johnston A. The Role of the Palatine Tonsils in the Pathogenesis and Treatment of Psoriasis. Br J Dermatol] 2012;18. doi: 10.1111/j.1365-2133.2012.11215.x.

[60] Nickoloff BJ. The immunologic and genetic basis of psoriasis. Arch Dermatol 1999;135:1104-1110.